Ask the Doctor

Herbs & Supplements
for Better Health

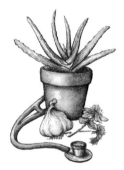

Derrick M. DeSilva Jr., M.D.

INTERWEAVE PRESS

Illustrations, Susan Strawn
Cover Design, Elizabeth R. Mrofka
Text copyright 1997, Derrick M. DeSilva, Jr.

INTERWEAVE PRESS
Interweave Press, Inc.
201 East Fourth Street
Loveland, Colorado 80537

Library of Congress Cataloging-in-Publication Data Applied For
DeSilva, Jr., Derrick M., 1957–

     Ask the doctor : herbs and supplements for better health
/ Derrick M. DeSilva, Jr.

     Includes resource directory and index
     ISBN 1-883010-31-4 : $12.95

Printed in the United States of America

First printing: 10M:397:OB

Dedication

To my loving and dedicated mother Mercedes and father Derrick, Sr., for the guidance and teaching me how to love.

To Father Richard Davis, T. O. R., for my Franciscan training.

To my boys Derrick, III, and Travis, whom I love so much that my heart smiles.

And last, but never least, my wife Susan, for putting up with me all these years.

ACKNOWLEDGEMENTS

I thank Linda Ligon and Logan Chamberlain of Interweave Press for their vision in encouraging me to write this book, and Doree Pitkin, book editor, for keeping me in line and keeping us on track.

PREFACE

My philosophy of medicine has its roots in Sri Lanka. We lived near the jungle, and my grandfather, Tatha, often took me along when he visited with his friends, many of whom were healers and religious people. Even at that early age, I enjoyed being around the jungle healers. They had an aura of wholeness; their very presence was comforting. Looking back, I believe that these individuals had cultivated an innate gift for healing, combining deep knowledge of people and folk medicine with a talent for observation and understanding.

At the age of nine I witnessed a healing of my father. When he was working in our garden one day, he came close to a nest where an old hen was sitting on her eggs. Alarmed, she rushed from the nest and pecked his leg, leaving a tiny wound. Soon a sore appeared. Even then we thought little about it, but the sore blew up into a horrible infection of the top layers of the skin.

Dad worked in the pharmaceutical industry then, and many of his friends were doctors who had access to the best medicines and therapies. Despite many efforts, Dad's sore didn't heal. Even a trip abroad to visit a respected specialist brought no results. The infection on his leg had destroyed an area of skin about eight inches square, and there seemed no way to stop it.

At last my grandparents suggested that one of the jungle doctors could help. Feeling he had nothing to lose, Dad trekked with Tatha through the jungle to the home of a local healer. When they returned, my grandmother, Aumma, boiled the many leaves they had been given for a poultice. We all vacated the house while the leaves simmered because they smelled so terrible. Every morning Aumma applied a poultice of the smelly stuff to Dad's leg. At the end of two or three weeks, we saw with amazement that the sore had completely disappeared, although it left a bad scar. My father, I'm thankful to say, is alive and well today, and the scar still reminds me of the Sri Lankan healers.

That experience galvanized me to become a doctor. I have never questioned that choice, or thought of another career. When we moved to Philadelphia, I attended a very formal, traditional school run by Franciscan monks. My college years were an amalgam of learning and fun, and in medical school I took on the additional challenge of becoming fluent in Spanish. I wanted to be a doctor who serves the health needs of many people, not only those who are easy to help.

After medical school, I spent over a year in research at a children's hospital and then completed my residency in internal medicine. On a trip to Florida to give a lecture on cardiovascular disease, I met a reporter for a major network, and we began to discuss our careers. I said, "Boy, I would love to do what you do."

"Why?", she asked.

"Instead of speaking to one person at a time," I replied, "I could speak to thousands of people at once."

The reporter suggested that I call my local radio station and offer to do a medical program. In my naivetè, that's what I did, and as luck would have it, the management of the station agreed. Thus my radio career began. It was lots of fun, and, as a young physician, I was seeing only ten patients a week, so I had plenty of time to devote to it. Now I see eighty to one hundred patients per week. The program is carried by Talk America Radio Network of Canton, Massachusetts, and currently reaches millions of people every week.

The people who call my radio show have taught me a good deal. In recent years, I've noticed a change in the questions they ask. Five years ago, a typical question was, "I have high blood pressure. I'm on a beta blocker and a diuretic. Do I have to take both? What do you think?"

Increasingly, I'm now asked a different kind of question. "I've just been diagnosed with high blood pressure. What can I do to control it, other than take medications?" Or, "I have high blood pressure. I'm taking medications, but I want to get off them. What can I do?"

To answer this new kind of question, I felt it necessary to talk about treatments outside the scope of conventional medicine—lifestyle changes, meditation, and natural nutritional and herbal therapies. To speak accurately and knowledgeably, I had to get busy and learn; medical doctors receive little or no training in the area of complementary medicine. I had one real advantage in my quest: My childhood experience in Sri Lanka had taught me that herbal medicine is valid. I had seen it heal my father, so I wasn't afraid to explore it. The more I looked into herbal medicine, and then other natural medicines, the more excited I became. Nowadays I share this knowledge, and my observations about the effects of natural medicine, in as many ways as I can.

Nonetheless, there is resistance to natural alternatives. There are rocks in the path of this new knowledge flowing down the stream, maybe a dam or two, but it is going to irrigate, nourish, and heal. While the medical community, as a whole, continues to resist, a few physicians have come to me saying, "I have the flu, and I really don't want to take antibiotics. Could you give me the name of something else that would help? What do you think about this echinacea stuff?" A cardiologist who heard me speaking about coenzyme Q10 asked me about it. One of the most respected eye surgeons in my area stopped me in the hall at the hospital to ask about bilberry after he heard me mention it on the radio. The radio program is generating interest among physicians, because their patients are asking them about natural treatments for ailments such as high blood pressure or diabetes. If that doctor doesn't know the answers, the patient will find someone who does. That possibility gets a doctor's attention.

Today, about half the American population has tried some form of alternative therapy such as herbs, vitamin supplements, acupuncture, massage, or homeopathy. Physicians can no longer say, "Here are your blood-pressure medications" and expect the patient to be satisfied—or, for that matter, to experience maximum health improvement. A better approach could be: "Here are your blood-pressure medicines, and you should also take garlic, coenzyme Q10, and hawthorn. And don't forget to to practice meditation and visualization." Today's patient benefits from the scientific, molecular approach to medicine, and from traditional healing, and from paying attention to the powers of the whole person. The results of this combination of approaches are superior to those of any one perspective.

This book is an attempt to capture the essence of the radio-program conversations that have stirred wide interest among my listeners and patients. Every call is fascinating in some respect—the question, the condition, the caller's tone of voice—but some more readily reflect the concerns of many, or stimulate informative discussions, or make an important point. I have selected questions of this sort from hours and hours of tapes, hoping to give the reader a lasting and helpful resource in seeking good health.

TABLE OF CONTENTS

How's Your Health?

Travis: "Dad, what can you wear any time that

never goes out of style?"

Father: "Hmm. I don't know, son, tell me."

Travis: "A smile, Dad!"

The body's most important function is to maintain homeostasis, a fine balance among its many organs and systems. This self-regulating and relatively constant state supports survival and growth. Illness is the disruption of homeostasis, and while illness persists we find it difficult to engage in our normal activities.

Conventional medicine today focuses on treating illness that has already occurred. While a few excellent examples of efforts to prevent illness have been developed by modern medicine—for example, programs to vaccinate young children against serious childhood disease—the overall approach is to treat active illness, and to do so using surgery and drugs. Insurance companies encourage this philosophy by failing to include annual physicals, vaccinations, and other preventive measures in their programs.

Missing from this picture is a thorough approach to preventing illness by promoting good health and supporting the body's ability to achieve and maintain it. More traditional approaches to medicine, generally termed alternative medicine, focus on stimulating the body's ability to heal itself, not destroying disease.

HOW'S YOUR ATTITUDE?

While in college, I kept a paper taped above my desk with "4.0" written on it. The paper represented my goal—to get perfect grades. I didn't reach that goal often, but I didn't waver from it. I visualized that grade on every paper, every exam, and every term report, and along the way I learned the power of visualization. Knowing clearly what you want and visualizing success in achieving it are important skills. I still use visualization to help achieve my goals, and I teach it to my children, believing that "If you shoot for the moon and miss, you'll hit the stars."

We can approach health issues in the same way. Bernie Siegel, author of several books on achieving health, says, "Visualize health, visualize feeling good." The mind can aid good health and healing, and the power of a smile, not only for those around you, but for your own body, is remarkable. Several reliable studies have shown that people who are smiling, happy, and jovial have more effective immune systems than those who are glum. Another study showed that people who are angry, bitter, or frustrated have higher incidences of heart disease and heart attacks than those who are generally happy.

I know that developing and maintaining a positive attitude isn't easy. I often have tough days, too. I've found that if I sit in my office for a little while, smile, close my eyes, do some deep breathing and some relaxation, I can restore a positive mental attitude. During such times, I think of the good things in life. If I'm feeling ill, I visualize my body healing and recovering. I soon return to work refreshed and able to continue with a smile.

In your quest for better health, use your mind to set the tone for your entire body. Improving your attitude and your outlook can be your first steps toward feeling better in every way.

THE DANGER OF DEPRESSION

Serious depression is the opposite of a positive mental attitude, and it frequently goes hand in hand with poor health. Does depression cause poor health, or does poor health cause depression? The answer to both questions is yes. Often unrecognized, depression disrupts the lives of millions by affecting diet, sleeping habits, behavior, relationships, thinking patterns, and the nervous system. Many studies have reported that people with depression are likely to become sick more often than others, and to recover more slowly. Depression's destruction of pleasure and hopefulness in life causes these patients to be more likely to engage in unhealthy habits. Untreated, depression can drag on for years.

Serious depression is more than feeling unhappy. Life's many disappointments and defeats cause sadness, sorrow, or grief. These useful emotions allow us to withdraw from the difficult situation and regroup, calm ourselves, and prepare to get on with life. Depression differs from sorrow in that is more intense than the situation requires and takes on a life of its own, disrupting basic brain chemistry and excluding the healing aspects of ordinary emotions.

Diagnosing Depression

Nationally, sixty percent of patients seen by physicians are depressed. Patients may complain of joint aches, poor concentration, fatigue, or weight gain, and their doctors may treat those symptoms although depression is the underlying problem. Even when patients clearly report depression, the physician, for whatever reason, may not take this seriously. The converse is also true; patients who report depression are sometimes handed a prescription for an antidepressant medication without a complete physical examination designed to expose illness that can cause serious depression. Neither situation is in the best interests of the patient.

Depression is not a simple case of the blues. Many physical conditions may cause depression. Hypoglycemia, allergies, thyroid disease, anemia, B_{12} and folic acid deficiencies are a few possibilities. Insufficient blood flow to the brain, such as occurs with hardening of the arteries, often causes the patient to feel depressed, anxious, and easily upset. Other possibilities are thyroid or pituitary imbalance, viral hepatitis, mononucleosis, and influenza. A thorough and knowledgeable physician will work with a depressed patient to rule out these conditions before treating the patient for depression.

The age-old stigma of mental illness may be one reason that both patients and physicians can be reluctant to deal directly with the issue of depression. We now understand this illness as a malfunction of brain chemistry that is often intertwined, at least initially, with a stressful and seemingly unsolvable problem that can range from a personal problem to forced repatriation in time of war. Like diabetes or an ulcer, depression is an illness that has causes, symptoms, and treatments.

Physicians, psychologists, and psychiatrists play important roles in the treatment of depression. Depressed patients typically face problems and issues that, despite a great deal of effort, they have been unable to solve. Psychologists are specifically trained to help such patients; the "talking cure" is extremely effective in resolving many of life's difficult issues. Psychiatrists are medical doctors who have intensively studied the physiology, chemistry, and manifestations of emotions and behaviors. Questioning, discussion, and medication are among the diagnostic and treatment tools of these physicians.

Treating Depression

I have observed that depressed patients who work with psychologists or other therapists *and* take medication seem to recover more quickly than those who rely on only one approach. Herbal medications are very effective in treating depression. St. John's-wort is very similar in its action to MAO inhibitors, popular and effective pharmaceutical antidepressants. A side effect of St. John's-wort is a higher tendency to sunburn. When anxiety is a component of depression, sedatives like valerian are often helpful. Omega 6 fatty acids are important, along with the B vitamins, calcium, and magnesium.

Other natural remedies treat the uncomfortable symptoms of serious depression. If you do not have high blood pressure, hypoglycemia, or a heart problem, you can try Siberian ginseng to increase your alertness. Kava kava counteracts the lethargy that plagues many depression patients. Melatonin, a natural hormone, can help depressive patients achieve more regular and healthful sleep when taken as directed.

Natural medicine also offers effective bodywork approaches to treating depression. Acupuncture, acupressure, and massage therapy are helpful in treating depression, especially if there are physical symptoms related to stress and tension. Regular exercise is also essential, because even moderate exercise releases endorphins, the body's pain relievers. Biofeedback techniques to cope with stress and anxiety are also very useful.

Diet also influences mood. Deficiencies of folic acid, zinc, selenium, and B_{12} have been implicated in depression. A diet that is high in vegetables and complex carbohydrates and low in fats supports balanced good health, and dietary supplements may help treat depression.

HOW'S YOUR DIET?

Many of us don't know how good, or bad, our food is. We know little about nutrition and are easily confused by dietary theories. As an example, consider the current concern about fat. Counting fat grams, counting fat exchanges, and investigating fat content is nearly a national obsession. Sales of low-fat and no-fat foods have skyrocketed. The truth, however, is that fat isn't bad; in fact, we need a certain amount of it for good health. But overindulging in fat makes us unhealthy.

Looking at the bigger picture, however, we must ask if the focus on eliminating fat reflects knowledge of good dietary principles. If we eat no fat but overeat breads and starches, will good health result? If we eat no fat but focus instead on eating mostly fruits, have we improved? No—a healthy balance among foods is necessary for a healthy diet.

Many people begin learning about nutrition and diet only after suffering a heart attack or other serious illness, yet nearly every community offers nutrition courses through community college or adult education programs, excellent magazines and books at the library or bookstore, or information through the American Heart Association or other service organizations. Learning about nutrition and good health earlier in life might head off those heart attacks and heart surgeries that motivate people to take their diets seriously. I believe that everyone should learn about good nutrition and health and apply that knowledge every day. We will be healthier, happier, and more productive if we do.

HERBAL MEDICINE

Humans have long used plants as both foods and medicines. Some of the healing tradition of plants has been lost or displaced by pharmaceutical medicine, but we are beginning to include herbs in a comprehensive approach to healing. To illustrate, in caring for a car, we must supply more than gasoline. Transmission fluid, brake fluid, and oil are needed as well. Similarly, our bodies need not only the care of physicians but herbs, vitamins, minerals, good food and water, and perhaps acupuncture, massage therapy, relaxation, and/or meditation. All these ways of caring for ourselves are important.

ON BEING A RESPONSIBLE PATIENT

Before you begin cutting lumber for your new deck, it's a good thing to carefully examine your plan. Improving your health with herbs and dietary supplements requires the same approach: educate yourself before leaping in. Knowledge of the basics will assist you in making appropriate decisions for yourself and in evaluating the outcomes of your choices. Without basic knowledge, you risk not only losing your money and time with useless products, but you might also damage your health.

Learning about herbs and dietary supplements is much easier today than it was only a few years ago. As the public has demonstrated greater interest in and acceptance of alternative forms of health care, publications and programs on the topic have become far more common. Many communities now have one or more stores specializing in these products, and public libraries are likely to carry numerous informative books and magazines. Support groups in the community focused around particular conditions may also be valuable. The local Yellow Pages may list alternative health practitioners who are available for consultation and guidance as well as treatments.

Better sources of information about alternative medicine will do much more than promote the particular form. Using herbalism as an example, a good magazine or book on the subject will include information about when NOT to use herbs, or when you should avoid an herb. Avoid those that overemphasize herbal medicine lore and select one that presents information based on research. If you find a book that tells you all the wonderful things about garlic—and it is wonderful —but none of the drawbacks, find a better source.

When taking herbs and dietary supplements, carefully follow the recommendations and dosages, particularly when using commercial preparations. These products are concentrated forms of the active ingredients of herbs, and exceeding the recommended dosage is very risky.

A knowledgeable health-store retailer is invaluable in helping you become familiar with products and companies with good track records. Ask if the firm belongs to the National Natural Food Association's Truth in Labeling program; those that do have pledged to accurately inform consumers about the contents of their products. I recommend that you always contact the company to ask for documentation on their products. If this is hard to get, do business with a company that is more cooperative.

In addition, metabolism varies greatly from one individual to another, so not everyone responds identically to a particular herb or dosage. In fact, as with pharmaceuticals, some don't respond at all to one herb or another. Fortunately, there's usually more than one way to solve any particular health problem, and another review of herbal information is likely to turn up another idea for treatment if one fails.

Reactions to herbs and dietary supplements are rare, but they can happen. For instance, people who are allergic to ragweed should avoid both echinacea and chamomile; these plants belong to ragweed's extended family and might provoke a respiratory reaction. More typically, patients come to me with diarrhea resulting from attempts to increase dietary fiber. Psyllium is an excellent dietary fiber, but if the body isn't used to a lot of fiber, severe diarrhea can result from taking too much. Our bodies need fiber, so I recommend that patients take half or even a quarter of the recommended dose and work up to a full dose over time. That is far better than abandoning efforts toward good health.

As herbs and dietary supplements become more popular, questions are being raised about the interactions of herbs and pharmaceutical medications. The answers to most of these questions are simply unknown; no research has been conducted. We do know certain facts—that vitamin E should not be used before surgery because it might cause excessive bleeding due to platelet activity, for instance—but the vast area of herbal interactions is largely unknown territory.

DEVELOPING A HEALING RELATIONSHIP

I believe that a physician is a healer, meaning that the physician seeks not only to heal the wound—the immediate problem—but to heal the whole person and empower the person as well. I try to teach patients the best route to improving their own health. The patient, however, must actually travel the road; I can't do that for her.

We can think of getting well as a trip through the woods. There are many hazards, and several possible routes. My job isn't to be the guide; my job is to point out the possibilities on the map. If she takes the river route, she needs to know there is white water near the bend, and she'll need a sturdy boat and life jacket. If she wants to travel the inland route, she'll find swamp, flies, and snakes, and she must prepare accordingly. By taking the long way, she'll find drought and slow going. It's not my place to direct the journey, but instead to point out the benefits and the pitfalls of each route. The traveler makes the final decision.

I believe that connecting with patients is essential, and even life-saving. A few months ago I met a 72-year-old patient at the emergency room because he was having chest pains. Joe is an unusual fellow because he plays a lot of tennis and, as he likes to remind me, he's a newlywed with a very active sex life. It just didn't seem right—why is this guy, who can play two sets of tennis without getting short of breath, suddenly having chest pains and panting when he walks up a flight of stairs?

Thinking back, I remembered that Joe had groin surgery several weeks prior. Perhaps he had developed a pulmonary embolism, a blood clot to the lung, despite the fact that this is rare once surgical patients are up and moving around. Pulmonary embolism, or PE, comes on suddenly and causes chest pain and shortness of breath.

The emergency room doctor who examined Joe didn't think my idea made any sense. The radiologist who I called out of bed in the middle of the night didn't agree, either. But when the tests were completed, there it was: a huge blood clot in the lung. If we had treated Joe for heart problems, he might have died, but instead he lived. So connecting with the physician who seeks to know you as a person is essential.

Doctors should put forth this effort, and patients, for their part, must be honest and open with the doctor. If you're taking ginseng or garlic or cayenne, your doctor needs to know it and for what purpose you are taking it, too. If you find that your doctor does not respect your efforts to improve your own health, find another doctor. You *must* have a physician who is willing to work with you and respect your point of view. Together, you and your physician *must* form the essential, central elements of your health-care team.

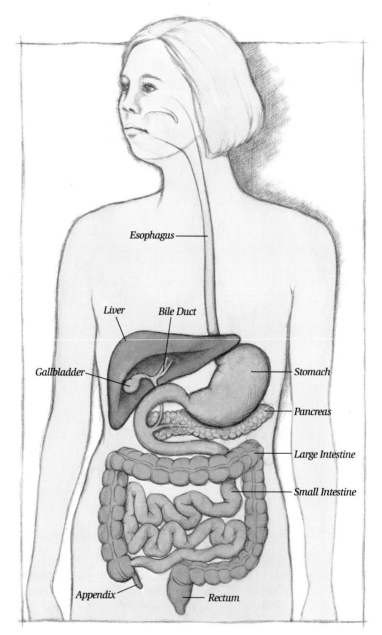

Esophagus —

Liver   Bile Duct

Gallbladder —   — Stomach

— Pancreas

— Large Intestine

— Small Intestine

Appendix —   — Rectum

The Digestive System

DIGESTION

Without good digestion,

good health is impossible.

Digestion is the complex process by which our food is converted into energy. It actually begins when we see and smell food and continues as we chew, mixing the food with saliva to begin the breakdown of carbohydrates. Acid is secreted in the stomach and contents are churned into a semiliquid that passes into the small intestine. Secretions from the liver, pancreas, and gall bladder reduce some compounds to molecules that pass through the wall of the small intestine into the bloodstream. The remaining compounds pass to the large intestine, which removes water and compacts the waste into stools that are excreted about 24 to 36 hours after eating. The kidneys also remove water and wastes from the blood stream and excrete them as urine. In the liver, nutrients are extracted and stored for future use; any excess is converted to fat.

We need many nutrients to keep the digestive system in good working order, and a basic balanced diet is the place to start. The greatest part of our food should be whole grains or whole-grain products, with smaller amounts of vegetables, fruits, eggs, meat, and very limited dairy products. Adequate water and fiber are necessary for proper digestion and elimination. Relaxation and exercise also contribute to digestive function.

Any sustained abdominal pain requires medical attention. Nationwide, ten percent of heart-disease patients first come to the doctor complaining of abdominal pain, unaware that they have heart trouble. Don't take a chance with abdominal pain—your stomach isn't likely to kill you, but your heart can so be careful.

See your doctor immediately if you find red blood in your vomit or stools. Also seek medical help if you pass a black, tarry stool. These symptoms can indicate serious problems; self-medication of any type is out of the question.

RELIEVING SOUR STOMACH

Q: What can relieve chronic sour stomach, other than antacids?
A: One of my favorite questions! For many years we believed that gastrointestinal problems, stomach problems, or sour stomach were caused by too much acid. So we treated these complaints by blocking acid with both prescription and over-the-counter antacids. Now we have new medications that completely shut off acid production. The problem is that acid is important. We can't digest our food without it. So this strategy may create more problems than it solves.

Treatment that builds the stomach's mucosal lining provides relief without compounding the patient's difficulties. Good acidophilus does this. In very stubborn cases, doctors can prescribe sucralfate, a medication that builds up the mucosa in the digestive tract. You should discuss treatment with your doctor.

ULCERS

Peptic ulcer disease includes both duodenal ulcers and gastric ulcers, sore places where the mucus lining of the stomach or intestine has become weak or absent, exposing stomach tissue to digestive acid. The duodenum is the top part of the intestine, and ulcers are common here; gastric ulcers appear lower in the stomach. Ulcer symptoms include abdominal discomfort, usually within an hour or two of eating and, typically, pain that interrupts sleep at 2 or 3 A.M., when the stomach is empty. The pain—sharp or dull or perceived as heartburn—is usually relieved by eating or swigging antacids. While ulcers are generally attributed to excess acid and/or pepsin, a large percentage are actually bacterial infections.

Other factors that can contribute to the development of ulcers are food allergies, lack of dietary fiber, stress, and smoking. The use of aspirin and nonsteroidal analgesics contributes to ulcer formation, too.

Diagnosing Ulcers

Q: My doctor says I may have an ulcer, and he took a blood test to make sure. I thought ulcers were caused by stress. What's this blood test all about?
A: Years ago everybody believed that stress caused ulcers, but that idea has now been questioned. Recent studies show that folks who get ulcers have no more stress in their lives than people who don't

> *Ninety percent of duodenal ulcers are caused by a bacteria, not stress.*

get them. In fact, ninety percent of duodenal ulcers are caused by a bacteria called *Helicobacter pylori,* or *H. pylori,* and a blood test can identify this infection. If you have it, antibiotics will eliminate it. Such medications destroy the bad bacteria like *H. pylori,* but they also destroy the good bacteria. To restore balance to the intestinal tract, take acidophilus, available from your health store.

Treating Ulcers

Q: Is there an alternative to the medications that totally shut off the stomach's acid production? My doctor says I might get an ulcer from having too much acid in my stomach, but it seems to me that stomach acid must serve some kind of purpose. At the same time I need relief from the stomach pain.
A: You're absolutely right! You need stomach acid for proper digestion, and most people don't think about that when they go to the doctor with stomach pain. They really hurt, and they're usually willing to take what the doctor prescribes as long as it relieves the pain. You're wise to question the medication.

We have two basic ways of treating ulcers. First, we can reduce the digestive acid that causes the burning sensation when it contacts the stomach or intestine, or we can thicken the mucosal lining of the digestive tract to protect the organs from the acid. The first strategy, unfortunately, disrupts digestion and can even cause cell changes in the digestive tract, but it is very popular nonetheless. Most people don't think about the fact that adequate digestive acid allows us to benefit from the foods we eat.

If the acid is decreased or shut off, problems can crop up in other areas. The second strategy, stimulating the mucosal lining to make it thicker and more protective, is better, I think. In this way we keep digestion in good order while protecting against ulcers.

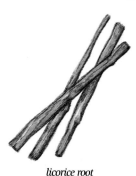

licorice root

Licorice for Ulcers

Q: I've heard that licorice works for ulcers, and that it's calming to the stomach. What do you think?

A: Licorice is soothing and good for ulcers, you're right about that. Of course I don't mean licorice candy because real licorice, the medicinal herb, is rarely used in candy. Medicinal licorice is the root of a plant that's been used for thousands of years to treat stomach problems.

Licorice is helpful in treating ulcers because it works against inflammation. It's also a mild diuretic and laxative, so it speeds the movement of matter through the system and helps remove toxins. Most importantly, it stimulates production of the mucosal lining, which protects the digestive tract, prevents ulcers, and supports healing.

If you have high blood pressure, a heart condition, or diabetes, be careful that your licorice is deglycerrhizinated; this form is often called DGL. Ordinary licorice makes you retain water and increases your blood volume, driving up your blood pressure. DGL stimulates the stomach's mucosal lining to make a thicker coating without side effects.

With these cautions in mind, it's good to take licorice to help ease ulcer pain. It's available in several forms; I prefer capsules, which are concentrated. You may prefer licorice tea, which is quite pleasant tasting as well as soothing.

CARING FOR THE LIVER

The liver, the largest organ of the body, weighs about four pounds. Bile, cholesterol, clotting factors, vitamin A, and complex proteins are manufactured by the liver; it also stores minerals, vitamins, and starch for emergency use. It filters out toxins and excretes them through the kidneys while regulating both protein metabolism and blood-sugar levels. Unique among the organs, the liver can regenerate up to twenty-five percent of its mass if it is injured or if part must be surgically removed.

Liver function can be disturbed by bacterial infection, alcohol, toxins, and structural problems. People with certain conditions such as alcoholism, diabetes, or those taking medications for seizure or chemotherapy can expect to develop liver problems. I recommend that these folks make special efforts to maintain liver health.

Liver Flush

Q: My health-nut friends insist that a liver flush would do me good. I don't know about this—my liver seems fine, and I'm a generally healthy person. They say they feel great after taking a liver flush.

A: Imagine a pretty fish tank with lots of colored fish in it, swimming here and there. Now look around the tank—is it fairly clean and healthy looking? Sure it is, because if it were dirty and unhealthy you couldn't see the fish, or the fish would be dead.

Now, imagine the aquarium filter. It's full of goo—algae, fish droppings, and other stuff that's been drawn out of the water. To keep the aquarium healthy, that filter has to be cleaned regularly.

The same applies to your liver, your body's filter. Toxins collect in the liver, and there are many toxins in our modern environments. The liver often needs help in eliminating them, and that's what a liver flush does—gives the liver a good cleaning and a boost.

Your body is like the aquarium. It's healthy and functioning well, but you probably ought to clean the filter to keep it that way.

Protecting the Liver

Q: I'm having a problem eating fatty foods like onion rings or fried chicken—and I love them. I get a burpy stomachache, sometimes even nausea. I don't eat these foods often, but I want to enjoy them when I do! Would a liver flush help?

A: Do you feel well otherwise?

Q: Sometimes I get gas pretty easily. I also have a problem keeping my energy up, although I do pretty well most of the time.

A: What kind of exercise do you like?

Q: None, actually. I walk a little, but I work at a computer all day. I don't have the chance for much exercise.

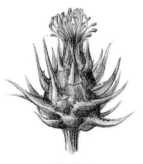

milk thistle

A: You would probably benefit from a liver flush. The fact that the fatty foods are causing you difficulty shows that your liver isn't able to digest the fats as it should. The gas goes along with that, too. And digestive upset saps your energy.

My first choice for a general liver cleanser is milk thistle, one of the best liver cleansers and protectors. Various commercial preparations are derived from the seeds. Milk thistle safely protects the liver by altering the cell structure of the outer membrane and helps it recover from damage by stimulating new cell growth. It is particularly effective against the damage of free radicals, alcohol, and other toxins.

Aloe vera gel also supports the liver. It softens the stools, eliminates toxins, and stimulates the immune system. It also encourages healthy bacterial flora in the intestine. The problem with aloe products today, however, is that many are primarily water. They are not concentrated enough to do much good. So take the time to find an aloe product that contains a high concentration of aloe gel and follow the directions.

Dandelion root, turmeric, and burdock root may also be helpful. Burdock root promotes perspiration—another way the body eliminates toxins—and thus helps the liver in its job. Another good cleanser for the liver is schisandra, an adaptogen used in Chinese herbology.

Now about that fried chicken: Give your digestive system a rest and don't eat any fatty foods for at least two months. Get the fat out of your diet, and concentrate on fresh foods and those low in fat and sugar. You'll see an improvement when, down the road, you try very small quantities of fried food as a portion of an otherwise healthy meal. If you're like a lot of other folks I've helped with this problem, one improvement will be that the greasy food doesn't taste so good any more—the healthier foods tastes much better.

Finally, you need to make some lifestyle changes and incorporate exercise into your routine. Start slow and work up; eventually you'll find that you have much more energy to do the things you like to do, and a great positive attitude. That will help you lose any excess weight as well, and you'll be healthier all around.

Hepatitis

Q: What is hepatitis?
A: Hepatitis is a serious liver disease that requires medical care. It can destroy the liver and cause death.

Q: How is it spread?
A: The most common form, hepatitis A, is caused by a virus and usually spreads by fecally contaminated food handled by someone who has the disease. The infection stimulates the body's immune system to form antibodies, which then protect from reinfection for life. Vaccines can guard against it for the same reason.

Hepatitis B, also viral, spreads by contact with infected blood. Monitors of the blood supply now test for hepatitis B, and we now see the disease most typically among drug users who share needles. Sometimes it's spread from mother to infant. Hepatitis B is tricky because a person can be contagious without showing symptoms.

Hepatitis C, once called non-A, non-B hepatitis, is similar to hepatitis B but becomes chronic more frequently. It is often discovered accidentally because sufferers often show few if any symptoms. The blood's antibodies against hepatitis C do not produce immunity.

Any inflammation of the liver can quickly become serious. Flu-like symptoms accompanied by yellowing of the skin, dark urine, and/or tenderness in the liver area require immediate medical attention.

ACIDOPHILUS AND DIGESTION

Acidophilus is a *probiotic,* a microorganism that is beneficial to human life. Without the many probiotics in our digestive systems—and elsewhere in our bodies—we could not live; some act to digest food, others to manufacture necessary nutrients, and still others to protect against infectious microbes that could cause illness. When correctly balanced, these rich colonies of microbes contribute to good health.

Acidophilus is an essential intestinal microbe that is available in several forms. Commercially prepared plain, live-culture yogurt contains beneficial strains of acidophilus, but it may also contain thickeners, sweeteners, and preservatives that detract from the healthful effects of the products. It is also made from processed cows' milk, which is one of the most common allergens. The best yogurt is that made at home from raw sheep's or goats' milk.

Preparations containing acidophilus can be purchased at your local health store in several forms. Capsules, especially enteric-coated ones that dissolve in the intestine, seem to be the most effective. Each product label includes recommended dosages and timing, and these should be followed. Acidophilus should always be refrigerated; if it gets too warm, it is no longer effective.

Several acidophilus strains are important: the DDS 1 strain, a normal inhabitant of the small intestine; the bifidobacter strain, which normally resides in the large intestine; and LB 51, a transient strain that lives throughout the intestines. When seeking an effective acidophilus product, select one that contains all three strains; each has a particular job to do in the body and together they're quite powerful. Sometimes patients report that they have some gas and digestive upset when they begin to take the acidophilus. If this happens, it's best to take only a half dose or quarter dose, and then work up to the full dose of acidophilus.

BOWEL PROBLEMS

Nineteen million Americans have digestive problems, so it's no wonder that related remedies are so heavily advertised today and frequently purchased. But using antacids and other such medications over a long period of time can lead to trouble for many, because the medications can disrupt the natural flora of the bowels and reduce the acid production necessary for good digestion and proper intestinal function.

There's nothing wrong with self-medicating *for a short time*, a week or less, but no longer. Now that acid-blocking medications such as Pepcid and Tagamet can be purchased over the counter, I'm worried that people will overmedicate themselves with these powerful drugs and mask symptoms. Folks with digestive problems could obtain better health by quitting smoking, caffeine, and alcohol; improving diet, and strengthening the mucosal lining of the stomach and intestines with deglycerrhizinated licorice and acidophilus.

Candida in the Digestive Tract

Candida albicans is a yeast-like fungus normally found in the intestine, genital tract, mouth, and throat. It usually lives in balance with other organisms, but it can overgrow and become a systemic problem. Because it infects many parts of the body, candida causes numerous symptoms.

Q: My system seems to produce too much acid. The acid builds up and then turns loose, and I get a problem with my plumbing: burning at the rectum and bladder discomfort. I drink only water and I eat well, but I do eat a good bit of bread.
A: Your symptoms indicate an overgrowth of yeast. First, cut down on the bread and eat only whole-wheat or multigrain products. These are much better for you than breads made from refined flour. I strongly suggest you use some acidophilus and cut the sugar from your diet.

Q: Is it true that candida is a normal inhabitant of the bowel that proliferates if you don't eat properly?
A: Yes. Candida is normally in balance with other bowel flora. Trouble starts when the good bacteria that assist digestion die from poor food, poor water, or the effect of birth-control pills, antibiotics, steroids, radiation, or chemotherapy. These factors do not target single cells but randomly destroy bacteria, allowing candida to flourish.

The overgrowth of candida in the digestive tract can cause real problems. Without the right bacteria in the digestive tract, the body becomes unable to use certain nutrients. This process is called malabsorption, and in my clinical practice I've seen it related to overgrowth of yeast.

A Plan for Overall Health

Q: My problem, first of all, is that I'm 81 years old.
A: That's not a problem!

Q: Thank you. I'm in generally good health, and I have routine check-

ups. *The only medication I take is for high blood pressure. But for a year or so, my mouth has been awfully dry. My lips, too.*
A: What medication do you take for your high blood pressure?

Q: It's a water pill.
A: That probably explains the dry mouth. Diuretics—water pills—drive water from the body, so sometimes we see that result. Do you have a coating on your tongue?

Q: No, I don't think so.
A: Tell me about your diet.

Q: I try to exclude candy, but I do eat sweets. And I love bread.
A: You probably have an overgrowth of candida or yeast in your mouth and digestive tract, even if you are not aware of any coating. Acidophilus will counteract it, and you probably should make some changes in your diet, too.

Begin slowly with acidophilus, and then work up. You should end up taking it both morning and at night, plus two more doses in the afternoon. As to your diet, eliminate sugar. Absolutely no candy, no cookies, no pie, no sugar in any form. That means, for at least one month, eliminate sugary treats, fruit, and fruit juices. When you shop for prepared food, read the label carefully to avoid hidden sugars; a good rule of thumb is that any ingredient ending in "ose" is a sugar.

Also reduce the bread and pasta. You could even stop eating all yeast products for the same amount of time. Refined, white flour is easily broken down into simple sugars during digestion, and this encourages the candida. If you eat cheese, eliminate that, too, because the microorganisms that form cheese could interfere with your digestion.

Q: Okay, I'll do it, but when should I see some results?
A: If you follow this plan conscientiously, by the end of six weeks you ought to see some results. A good program takes at least that long to bring your flora into balance.

Q: I wish I'd learned about this sooner.
A: That's a very good point. But it's never too late—it's absolutely never too late make a change and do the right thing.

It's never to early, either. Nearly every child aged 8 or 9 can grasp the basic principles and understand the importance of nutrition. They can also learn about simple, helpful remedies. As individuals and as a nation, good health is so important that I believe health and nutrition should be taught in every school in the United States.

Malabsorption

Q: How do you know if you have malabsorption?
A: Malabsorption causes dry skin, tiredness, and sometimes depression, gas, weight loss or gain, and constipation or diarrhea. These symptoms are shared with numerous other ailments, so it is best to get a good diagnosis that rules out other problems if these symptoms occur.

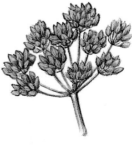

fennel seed

Malabsorption often responds to treatment with acidophilus and digestive enzymes such as papain. The herbs ginger and peppermint, which calm the stomach and ease intestinal spasms, may help as well. Fennel seed is also calming and soothing to the stomach.

One more word on malabsorption. Some believe it's related to aging, but I believe it results from damaging the intestines with toxins, stimulants, and chlorinated water. I'm not opposed to chlorine in the water, but the chlorine should be filtered out of the water before it is used. Numerous home water filters effectively remove chlorine and other substances.

Intestinal Upset

Q: I seem to get intestinal upsets, possibly food poisoning, rather easily. Is there any way I can avoid this problem?
A: You can prevent some episodes by maintaining the flora of your intestinal tract. When the intestine is thoroughly coated with acidophilus, as is normal, salmonella or other harmful bacteria cannot attach. They are automatically eliminated from your system, causing little or no problem. Also, you can promote good organisms by avoiding sugar and refined flour, which encourage the growth of bad organisms by breaking down into simple sugars. When you maintain the right balance of intestinal

flora, bad food or water may give you some subtle symptoms, gas or discomfort maybe, but you'll avoid diarrhea. You can prevent a lot of what we call intestinal flu by eating well, drinking good water, and cultivating the protective intestinal organisms.

Gastroesophageal Reflux Disorder

Q: If I take acidophilus, will that get rid of my GERD—gastroesophageal reflux disorder?

A: No, GERD is something else altogether, although it feels a lot like sour stomach and other kinds of heartburn. Basically, GERD is a leaky valve between the stomach and the swallowing tube, the esophagus. The bad valve lets digestive acid leak up into the esophagus, and it hurts.

To cope with GERD, I recommend that patients use deglycerrhizinated licorice to stimulate new growth in the mucosal lining of the digestive tract. They should also quit all the bad habits, like cigarettes, alcohol, and caffeine, that stimulate excess stomach acid production.

Two other suggestions really help. Raise the head of your bed with a board or bricks; the acid, a liquid, follows gravity, and that's why people with GERD have discomfort when they sleep. With the head of the bed raised, the acid stays in the stomach. And don't eat anything for at least one, and preferably two hours before bedtime. You'll find that your discomfort is far less if you follow these suggestions.

Irritable Bowel Syndrome

Q: What exactly is irritable bowel syndrome? From what my doctor said to me, after all kinds of tests, it means that I'm perfectly healthy except I have constipation and diarrhea all the time, and the doctor can't figure it out.

A: Irritable bowel syndrome (IBS) is quite mysterious and frustrating because we don't understand it well at all. But I'm glad you've had all those tests because IBS symptoms are very similar to those of diverticular disease, parasites, and cancer, among others. The tests eliminate these possibilities.

The typical patient is a busy, meticulous woman aged 20 to 40. Her gastrointestinal tests are negative but she still reports a painful abdomen, usually the lower right quadrant, and diarrhea and/or constipation. Some think that the colonic nerves of IBS patients spasm painfully in an abnormal reaction to stimuli such as stress or certain foods. There are other theories, too. Everyone agrees, however, that IBS does not lead to problems like cancer or ulcerative colitis. So that's good news!

Q: It would be good news for me if I could get control of this problem. What can I do?
A: Let me ask you a couple more questions. Do you have a lot of stress in your job or personal life?

Q: I guess so. I'm a single mother, and I work the night shift as a police dispatcher. I'm also working for a promotion and a raise.
A: Are you allergic to anything?

Q: I don't think so. I've never had an allergic reaction.
A: Okay. So it sounds like you have a lot of stress, but no allergies. With IBS, what works with one individual doesn't work with another, but I do suggest that you first tackle the stress. Relaxation techniques are often taught at community centers and community colleges; see if you can find a class in yoga, meditation, or biofeedback, or get some books at the library and teach yourself. Many cases of IBS go hand in hand with depression and clear up when the depression is treated. So talk to your doctor about that possibility as well.

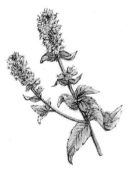

peppermint

Further, slowly increase the fiber in your diet and be sure to include a rich variety of vegetables. Drinking chamomile tea may help, as this herb acts as an antispasmodic for the bowel. Rosemary, peppermint, and balm teas help as well. Some report that enteric capsules of peppermint oil that dissolve in the intestine are effective. And be sure to take acidophilus, which ensures that the good bacteria and the bad bacteria in your bowels are well balanced.

To determine your best treatment, however, I recommend that you keep a "food and feelings" diary for at least two months. Every day, record what you are eating and your emotional state, when you have an IBS attack, the symptoms, and anything else that seems pertinent, like a particularly pleasant or stressful event. This careful recording may reveal a pattern of IBS attacks related to a food you are eating, to stress, to a particular emotional state, or to some other factor. Once you find that out, you'll be on the road to addressing the root of your IBS.

Lactose Intolerance

Q: I am completely lactose intolerant so I'm concerned about getting an adequate amount of calcium. What is your recommendation? I'm a woman, 53, on hormone replacement therapy. Is it possible to become lactose tolerant again?

A: Yes, that is possible. Since you are lactose intolerant, I assume you have some stomach problems. Do you take a lot of antacids?

Q: No, I don't.

A: That's good. There's a debate in the medical community right now about whether to block stomach-acid production. I say our bodies need that acid to digest food properly. In my practice I recommend building up the body's mucous lining to protect tissues from the acid, which is necessary to digestion, rather than block it.

First, make sure you don't have a *Helicobacter pylori* infection, which causes ulcers and abdominal pain, or some other abdominal problem. The symptoms of lactose intolerance—abdominal discomfort, flatulence, and diarrhea—are the symptoms of other illnesses as well, so it can be confusing. Get an accurate diagnosis for your abdominal pain.

Then, make sure your system has enough acidophilus, which helps your digestion and will ease your symptoms. The acidophilus allows the right bacteria to grow in your intestine. You digest food more efficiently, and any irritating substance that passes through your system will give you less trouble.

Acidophilus won't cure your lactose intolerance, but the intensity of your reactions will be less if you take it. In the meantime, try some of the dairy alternatives such as rice milk or soy milk, or even some of the special milk products that have the lactose removed or reduced.

As for your calcium intake, you can do two things. First, use a form of calcium that is soluble and easy to digest, such as calcium citrate, calcium gluconate, or calcium phosphate, especially if you are menopausal or past menopause. These forms are available as liquids, and I like them because they make less work for the stomach. Studies show that women past menopause have very little stomach acid compared to younger people; that means they can't digest the most popular form of calcium supplement, calcium carbonate.

> *Women past menopause need a calcium supplement that is easy to digest.*

Magnesium is essential to the absorption of calcium, and you may want to try that, too. Also be sure that you are getting enough of the vitamins B_6 and B_{12} and vitamin D. Moderate exercise, such as brisk walking, for one hour, three times per week, also helps prevent bone loss.

Crohn's Disease

Q: What is Crohn's disease?
A: Crohn's disease is a painful intestinal inflammation, usually involving the large intestine. Patients typically feel pain in the lower right abdomen, and they usually report bloating and bloody stools. Diagnosis is made by colonoscopy and biopsy of the mucosa. Under normal conditions, the inside of your intestine looks like the inside of your cheek: smooth, pink, and healthy. If you have Crohn's disease, however, your intestine is inflamed, sore-looking, and sometimes even bleeding. Although Crohn's disease is not rare, nobody really knows what causes it.

Crohn's disease may be caused by an autoimmune disorder, in which the body attacks itself; there may be a genetic factor; or perhaps it is caused by an undetected infectious agent. Personally, I think that Crohn's disease is somehow involved with leaky gut syndrome, in which molecules of undigested proteins pass through the wall of the intestine and start the immune response.

Q: Yuck! What happens then?
A: Well, imagine that you want to water your lawn and you grab your soaker hose instead of your regular hose. Both hoses look alike, but when you turn the water on, droplets of water seep from the hose surface. You have the wrong hose.

Now think of your intestine as the hose. You want the regular one that carries its contents from one place to another, but instead it's leaking through its surface. As molecules that are not digested or absorbed seep out of the intestine, the body identifies them as invaders and attacks them. Soon the intestine itself is inflamed.

To treat Crohn's disease, be very careful with diet. I'm sure your doctor has told you to cut out alcohol, caffeine, and tobacco in any form. You ought to be eating a diet very high in fresh vegetables that are low in acid, such as broccoli, carrots, celery, spinach, cabbage, and kale. Eliminate meat and dairy products. Don't eat fried food, either, because fat is difficult to digest and can irritate the colon. You must have plenty of good, fresh water. Cabbage juice is an excellent healer.

Q: Can't steroids cure Crohn's disease?
A: We often treat Crohn's disease with steroids such as prednisone. While I believe that steroids can perpetuate the problem and even make it worse, it does happen that a patient with an acute condition needs fast-acting therapy. A short course of steroids gets right to the inflammation, which produces the pain, and the patient gets relief. I recommend against long-term use of steroids because they can cause osteoporosis, cataracts, and lots of candida. They also suppress the immune system.

Over the long run, I believe that herbal remedies aimed at healing the intestinal lining are best. Acidophilus has this effect, of course, and it also reduces gas, bloating, and discomfort. Papain, an enzyme present in unripe papaya and available in commercial preparations, breaks down proteins, making the intestine's job easier. High-fiber supplements such

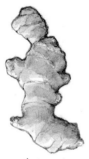

ginger root

as psyllium husks add bulk. In addition, the soothing and healing herbs such as ginger, aloe vera gel, and licorice can be taken to promote internal repair. Good water, of course, is important, as are the B vitamins.

Diverticulosis
Q: What is diverticulosis?
A: Imagine the intestine as a tube with various elastic properties. Now imagine that you blow up

a tiny plastic glove so the fingers stick down into that tube. The tiny fingers are the diverticulae in the intestine, and they usually develop at weak sites where veins enter the colon. They are big enough to be seen by the naked eye or on an X-ray; they're also big enough to cause trouble. Any foods that aren't easily digestible get caught in these fingers and putrefy. An inflammation develops, and the patient gets a low-grade fever, pain typically in the left lower part of the belly (as opposed to the right lower quadrant, where the appendix is), and generally doesn't feel well.

Q: Can I get rid of diverticulosis? Do I have to have surgery?
A: If the diverticulae rupture, the intestinal contents will leak into the abdominal cavity and cause peritonitis, which is a very serious and possibly life-threatening condition. If your doctor is talking about surgery for diverticulosis, you may have one of the very serious cases that requires surgery.

Q: No, my doctor didn't say I need surgery. But a friend did have surgery, and it was hard on her.
A: All surgery is hard, and it's best to do everything you can to avoid it. If you have a typical case of diverticulosis, start now with a bulky, high-fiber diet to reduce pressure in the intestine. Make sure you drink plenty of good water.

When stools are dry, hard, or compacted, they are difficult to pass and create pressure in the large intestine, contributing to the development of diverticulae, and probably hemorrhoids, too. This is why we ought not to strain when moving the bowels. A diet high in fiber softens the stools by increasing their bulk and water content so they pass more readily. People who are sensitive to roughage can try water-soluble fibers such as pectin or oat bran. Some other things that are helpful include the enzyme papain, peppermint leaves, and ginger.

Q: Will doing this clean out my intestine?
A: It will help the problem, but it won't change the anatomy of the intestine. Preventing inflammation is the best course.

Regularity
Q: I'm 41 years old, in very good health, run marathons, and eat as well

as I can. But I travel a lot, so for the past two years I've been taking psyllium fiber.
A: How much psyllium fiber do you take?

Q: *About a quarter of a cup in the evening, mixed with water.*
A: Psyllium husk is a tried and true fiber that promotes elimination; it is mucilaginous and produces bulk. I think you should check with a gastroenterologist, though, because you've been taking quite a lot of psyllium over a long period.

Follow the directions carefully when you are taking psyllium or any other herbal product. A typical psyllium dose is a couple of teaspoons in a glass of water after every meal. Some have success with aloe vera gel.

Don't worry about psyllium or other natural laxatives washing away nutrients from your body. They're quite safe. But if you find yourself suffering from constant constipation, you need to see a gastroenterologist for a complete evaluation.

GIARDIA AND CRYPTOSPORIDIA

Q: *I'm waiting for the results of a parasite test that my doctor ordered because I have abdominal pain and really embarrassing gas. I don't know whether to be insulted or not. I keep myself clean, and I thought only people with poor hygiene got tapeworms and stuff like that.*
A: Parasites are more common than people think. Anyone can get them, even with excellent hygiene, because raw fruits and vegetables or even tap water carry parasites. Your doctor is probably on the lookout for the microscopic parasites cryptosporidia and giardia, both increasingly common in the water supply, particularly in private well water. These parasites are not detected by most water purity tests and pass through most water filters.

Crypto causes fatigue, diarrhea, and abdominal pain. Antidiarrheal medications aggravate it, and no medications now known can eliminate it. The best thing to do is conscientiously replace fluids lost to the diarrhea and wait out the infection, usually a couple of weeks. You may try ginger or peppermint to ease the symptoms.

Giardia is a different story. People usually get it from fecally contaminated water—drinking from clear, beautiful mountain streams while camping is a classic example, because wildlife carry it—or from unprotected sex. Giardia causes abdominal pain, extreme gas, and bad-smelling, floating stools; fortunately, antibiotics destroy it.

While most people infected with these parasites suffer a period of misery before recovering, others may die. Remember the cryptosporidosis outbreak in the Milwaukee area several years ago? About 100 people died from drinking contaminated public water. This was a real wake-up call to America to clean up public water supplies. I also noticed that nearly everyone who died in Milwaukee had a suppressed immune system. That is, they were undergoing chemotherapy or radiation therapy, or had AIDS or another illness that interfered with their immune system, and the parasitic infection overwhelmed them. Anyone with such a condition should be very, very careful to avoid parasitic infections.

Q: If there are parasites in the public water supplies, what can we do to protect ourselves? Should we all be buying bottled water?

A: Bottled water is no solution. Because bottled water is completely unregulated, you have no assurance that it is superior in any way to your tap water. If you like it, that's okay, but it's not necessarily an improvement over your tap water.

You *can* protect yourself against giardia and cryptosporidia by careful hygiene—I know you are already conscientious about that—and by washing your hands frequently. Be sure to thoroughly wash all your fruits and vegetables, too. The best thing, however, is to invest in a home water filter system that uses a one-micron filter to remove contaminants from your water. It captures those tiny little cryptos and the giardia, too. Maintain the filter carefully and it will be your best protection.

> *Bottled water may not be an improvement over your tap water.*

In addition, you can start yourself on a course of acidophilus. A strong intestinal coating of this good bacteria prevents parasites from causing a lot of trouble in the digestive tract. Acidophilus has many other benefits as well. Given your symptoms, I think it will help you.

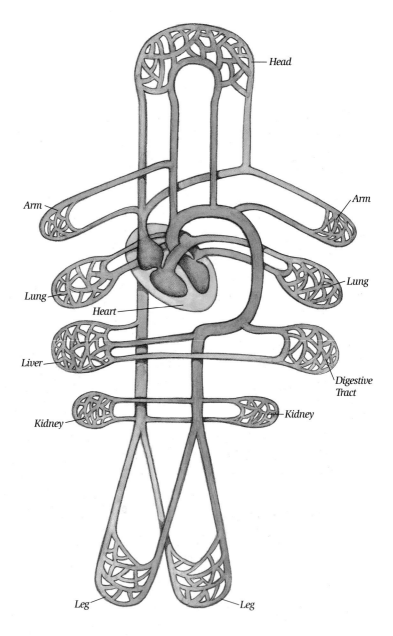

The Circulatory System

How's Your Heart?

Every thirty-two seconds, an American has a heart attack.

Heart disease remains our number one killer.

Every year, one million Americans die from cardiovascular disease, the leading cause of death in the United States. Fifty million more suffer from cardiovascular problems, and many don't know it because they are without symptoms. Heart disease is so common, in fact, that many believe age and cardiovascular problems go hand in hand. Although cardiovascular disease is much more common among older people, the illness is not inevitable.

Some factors that increase the chances of heart disease can be controlled. Diabetes, high blood pressure, and high cholesterol, put you at risk. Smoking, overweight, and lack of exercise hurt the heart. Too much stress, too much coffee and alcohol, and too little relaxation all contribute to the process of heart disease, too. Serious heart damage results from our modern diet, which is typically full of refined sugar and flour, high in fats, and low in dietary fiber.

Some factors can't be controlled. If your family history includes heart disease, or if one of your parents had a heart attack before the age of 55, your chances of heart disease increase. If your high blood pressure is hereditary, you may find it very difficult to control.

An honest examination of your individual habits and situation can lead to improved cardiovascular health. Years ago when Dr. Dean Ornish first published his book on reversing heart disease, the medical community laughed at him. Now his work is well respected.

Ask yourself these questions: Are you controlling your blood pressure and keeping it within normal limits? Does your diet include lots of fruits and vegetables, whole-grain products, and little red meat, eggs, and dairy products? How about exercise—do you walk or bike or swim at least three times a week at a moderate rate? Is your weight normal for your sex, height, and age? If you are diabetic, do you control your blood sugar appropriately? Are you a smoker? Each of these factors are within individual control, yet many prefer to overlook the facts, maintaining, "Heart problems go along with old age. The old ticker just wears out."

CHOLESTEROL AND HEART HEALTH

Cholesterol is necessary for good health and normal function. It's essential to nerve function, the production of sex hormones, and other bodily processes. However, the liver generates all the cholesterol the normal body needs, and we make trouble for ourselves when we take in additional cholesterol through a fatty diet or consume sugar or alcohol, both of which stimulate the liver's cholesterol production. Cholesterol is implicated in heart disease; it forms the plaque that clogs arteries and can lead to heart attacks.

Q: I'm not even 40 yet and my doctor says I have high cholesterol. Does that mean I'm going to have a heart attack? Also, my doctor mentioned several kinds of cholesterol. That confused me.
A: What is your cholesterol level?

Q: He says it's 236. I thought you didn't have to worry until it hit 300, and 236 would be low.
A: Your ideal cholesterol level is related to your age, and you should ask your doctor the best way to calculate it for yourself. I think a cholesterol level of 236 is higher than average for your age, and you need to work to push that down to under 200.

Regardless of age, when you hit 240 your risk of coronary heart disease shoots up. At 300, people have a very high incidence of heart attacks. You are in a range where you can do a lot to prevent yourself from developing serious cardiovascular problems.

Your doctor probably was talking about the three main types of cholesterol. Low-density lipoprotein (LDL) is the "bad cholesterol" that packs itself into the blood vessels, causing atherosclerosis and heart attacks. The LDL level should be 120 to 130. The "good" cholesterol is high-density lipoprotein (HDL), which attaches to other fat molecules and actually removes them from the system through the intestine, lowering total cholesterol and perhaps even removing LDL cholesterol from the walls of the arteries. The HDL level should be between 45 and 50. Finally, the very-low-density lipoprotein (VLDL) carries the triglycerides, which play an important role in fat metabolism; the triglyceride level should be 140 to 150.

In the long run, your total cholesterol number is useless; instead, you should know your separate HDL, LDL, and triglyceride levels. The critical number is the ratio of total cholesterol to HDL; it should be 4 or less. Generally, total cholesterol count should be less than 200, and HDL should be between 45 and 50. If you have a total cholesterol of 200, and you divide that number by your HDL level—suppose it is 50—the ratio is 4, the maximum number. At that point, you should make efforts to decrease your total cholesterol count.

Q: How do I do that, besides eliminating meat, dairy, and egg products from my diet and getting some exercise?
A: You should do those things for sure, but there are other factors that you can't control. Men get more heart disease than women, and high cholesterol runs in some families. If that's your case, you may need medication along with other steps that lower your risk of heart attack.

The American Heart Association recommends that your diet be made up of no more than thirty percent fat, with ten percent or less coming from meat, eggs, dairy products, and so on. Losing excess weight often has a big impact on cholesterol. Are you fairly relaxed?

Q: I think of myself as ambitious and energetic guy, but my wife's nickname for me is "Type A."
A: You should evaluate your outlook and response to various situations. Type A people tend to overreact to situations, and they're always in a hurry. They never have enough time, and they're often hostile and aggressive. Does that sound like you?

Q: Well, sometimes, yeah.

A: One set of studies tells us that Type A folks have more heart attacks than more easy-going people. That's the bad news. Another set says that Type As survive their heart attacks more often than the easy-going Type Bs. That's the good news. But not too good, because a third of first-time heart attack victims die.

I recommend that you start lowering your stress level and learn some relaxation techniques like meditation or biofeedback. This will help you control your reactions and stay calm. And get exercise. Exercise not only stimulates your cardiovascular system but also reduces stress and gives most people a more positive outlook. All these things working together can help lower your cholesterol and keep you healthy.

Apart from diet and exercise, several herbs and supplements are helpful for reducing cholesterol levels. Hawthorn is probably one of the best herbs for cardiovascular problems in general because it lowers both cholesterol and blood pressure while slowing the heartbeat and strengthening the heart's pumping action.

Gugulipid, an extract of the resin of the mukul myrrh tree, stimulates the liver to metabolize LDL cholesterol. Research shows that elevated cholesterol levels in humans dropped 14 to 27 percent and triglycerides drop 22 to 30 percent when gugulipid is used. Side effects are minimal or none.

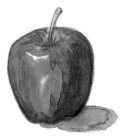

apple

Apple pectin is an excellent substance for lowering cholesterol. Its fiber intercepts the cholesterol secreted by the liver and carries it out of the system.

Q: So how many apples a day should I eat?

A: I guess an apple a day will still keep the doctor away, but don't peel it! The apple peel contains a lot of fiber. Psyllium husk is also high in soluble fiber and carries cholesterol out of the body.

HIGH BLOOD PRESSURE

High blood pressure, or hypertension, is the silent killer. It's the major cause of heart disease and the number one cause of strokes in this country, and it can also damage the eyes, kidneys, and blood vessels. Yet most people don't know they have it until they're in serious trouble, because high blood pressure usually has no symptoms until it's quite advanced. The incidence of high blood pressure rises with age. Half of all Americans 55 and older have high blood pressure, rising to 63 percent after age 65. Three-fourths of African-Americans over 65 have it. While high blood pressure does run in families and it's strongly correlated with obesity, the root cause in most cases remains unknown.

So while we don't know exactly what causes high blood pressure, we do know its effects. Stroke is the most dreaded; hypertension can also cause headaches, deterioration of vision, difficult breathing, congestive heart failure, and kidney failure. Hypertension is a devastating disease, but mild to moderate cases can be managed successfully using many of the same approaches that promote overall heart health and lower cholesterol.

Measuring Blood Pressure

Q: How do blood-pressure machines actually work?
A: It measures the blood vessel's resistance to the blood going through it. Your doctor listens to the pulse inside the elbow and pumps the cuff up until it turns off the pulse. Then he deflates the cuff until he hears the first sound, which is the top number, and listens until the last sound stops, and that's the bottom number.

The definition of high blood pressure is resistance to flow. For example, think of a gallon of water flowing through a tube six inches in diameter. Now, try to send that same gallon of water through a tube that is only three inches in diameter. The small tube has a greater resistance to flow and produces a higher pressure. Similarly, high blood pressure means that the blood vessels are narrowed in some way and resist the flow of blood.

The degree of resistance is expressed as measurements of systolic pressure, taken when the heart is at rest, or full of blood; and diastolic pressure, taken when the heart contracts and pumps blood into the arteries. Regardless of age, the systolic pressure, which is expressed first, should be under 140, and the diastolic pressure between 85 and 88.

Q: *Are the blood pressure monitors in supermarkets and drug stores reliable?*
A: Usually. In some parts of the country, however, there has been controversy about their accuracy. If you have doubts, ask the pharmacist about whether his machine is regularly checked and calibrated for accuracy.

Q: *How often should blood pressure be checked, and when is it usually the highest?*
A: If you are on blood pressure medication, check your blood pressure readings at least three to five times a week. Your blood pressure will be higher in the morning. While we are sleeping, about 3:00 or 4:00 A.M., our bodies start to secrete hormones to prepare us for awakening. These hormones, called catecholamines, also narrow the blood vessels, so the blood pressure goes up when they kick in. I advise my patients to take their blood-pressure medications before bed. The peak effect will occur when they are waking up in the morning, counteracting their highest blood pressure.

Q: *I've heard that Monday is heart-attack day. Is that true?*
A: Yes. To be even more precise, Monday morning at 9 A.M. Why? You're nervous, you're anxious, you've got to get busy after a weekend off. So the most dangerous day of the week is Monday, and the most dangerous time of the day is between 6 and 10 A.M.

Treating High Blood Pressure
Q: *What medications help high blood pressure?*
A: Remember that troublesome three-inch tube we talked about? It was too narrow to easily handle the gallon of water we tried to pour through it. When prescribing drugs to treat high blood pressure, we can use one of two basic medical strategies. We can expand the tube for easier flow by opening up the blood vessels or we can pour less liquid through the tube by reducing volume, thus reducing flow.

For the first strategy, we can prescribe alpha blockers or angiotensin-converting enzyme (ACE) inhibitors to block hormones that narrow the blood vessels. Calcium channel blockers also allow the blood vessels to dilate by preventing calcium-dependent contractions of the vascular muscles. These blockers are prescribed for angina and certain kinds of heart arrhythmias. Other vasodilators also lower the blood pressure by relaxing the muscles of the blood vessels.

For the second strategy to lower blood pressure, we prescribe diuretics or water pills that eliminate excess fluids from the system. This eases the heart's job.

Patients who begin taking blood-pressure medications—especially beta blockers—should not stop taking them without their doctor's approval. If these medications are discontinued, the blood pressure can shoot up again, maybe higher than ever, with serious consequences.

Q: I've been prescribed calcium-channel blockers, but since I'm in my fifties and past menopause, I'm concerned about osteoporosis. Do calcium-channel blockers counteract my calcium supplements?
A: No, not at all. These medications do not affect the bones or their function, nor do they prevent the bones from receiving the calcium. They work in an entirely different way, so you don't need to worry about taking the prescription.

Q: I've been prescribed diuretics to lower my blood pressure. Is there anything else I should be doing?
A: Diuretics are often prescribed to help lower blood pressure, but you can lose significant amounts of minerals like potassium, calcium, and magnesium while you are taking them. Then you can develop problems with poor appetite, nausea, weakness, and drowsiness.

Ask your doctor for a diuretic that does not drain the potassium from your body. Take a good multivitamin, and eat plenty of bananas, citrus fruits, tomatoes, potatoes, legumes, deep yellow vegetables, and some meat. Include calcium-fortified foods such as orange juice with calcium added, and green, leafy vegetables. For magnesium, the green leafy vegetables are again good, and so are whole grains, nuts, soybeans, and seafood. All in all, eat a good diet high in fruit, vegetables, and fiber.

Lowering Blood Pressure
Q: Are there any herbs that I can take to help lower my blood pressure?
A: My favorite alternative therapy for lowering high blood pressure is garlic. If you can eat raw garlic—three to five cloves per day—without

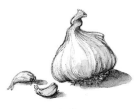

garlic

developing digestive problems, that's great. To use garlic in a commercial preparation, make sure the allicin content is high so you get a strong dose, and enteric capsules that dissolve in the intestine are best. Some products also have the garlic odor removed, and many people prefer those. All in all, garlic is excellent for heart problems, lowering blood pressure, and lowering triglycerides. One caution about garlic, however, is that it interferes with blood clotting. So if you are taking Coumadin to prevent clotting, or if you anticipate surgery, don't eat a lot of garlic. It may make your blood too thin.

Because you're interested in using herbs to lower your blood pressure, I want to warn you to avoid ephedra or its relatives like pseudoephedrine. Sometimes these herbs are called ma huang and used in Traditional Chinese Medicine (TCM). It's commonly used in cold medicines, and it's great for preventing bronchiospasm, but it drives up blood pressure. Heart beat speeds up and sometimes becomes irregular, and dizziness and nervousness are also side effects. You don't need any of that—so stay away from ephedra.

Low Blood Pressure

Q: Every so often I feel tired and worn out for no good reason. I have no other symptoms. I just feel worn out.

A: If you feel lethargic and groggy for no particular reason, you may have low blood pressure. In general, the lower your blood pressure, the better, unless symptoms like yours are evident. Nearly identical symptoms show up in chronic fatigue syndrome. I ask patients with that problem to drink eight glasses of water a day along with a pinch of salt; this raises the blood pressure and helps them feel a bit better. You can do the same when your blood pressure is low—increase your water consumption and throw a pinch of salt in two or three of those glasses of water.

Erratic Blood Pressure

Q: My blood pressure varies a lot, from very low to quite high.

A: Erratic blood pressure can indicate a rare condition called pheochromocytoma, which affects only one or two percent of those with high blood pressure. Pheochromocytoma is an abnormal but usually benign growth on the adrenal gland that secretes various hormones and chemicals rather randomly, driving the blood pressure up rapidly. It is a rare condition, and the diagnosis is made by measuring the patient's catecholamine levels and analyzing urine tests. Treatment involves ACE inhibitors or surgery.

You should certainly avoid the stimulant ephedra and related chemicals such as pseudoephedrine; these will make your high blood pressure higher yet, which is not good. Look for these ingredients in any over-the-counter cold medicines.

Preventing High Blood Pressure

Q: How can I change my diet to protect against high blood pressure? My mother died of a stroke and my father had hypertension. I don't want to have that kind of trouble.
A: Is your doctor worried about your blood pressure?

Q: No, I'm just 28 and it's normal now. But I do want to stay healthy.
A: That's a very good attitude. Has anyone mentioned familial hypertension to you? Some folks, regardless of their diet, weight, exercise, and so on, have a strong genetic predisposition to hypertension, and they can't help it. People with this condition must be more diligent with their diet and general health care than others. At some point, they may need medication.

Since you haven't developed high blood pressure yet, you might consider cayenne, or capsicum. It helps lower blood cholesterol and prevent blood clots. Cayenne is also believed to normalize blood pressure; that is, it raises blood pressure that is too low and lowers blood pressure that is too high. Some new cayenne preparations are not so fiery tasting as the older ones. Hawthorn is also an excellent herb for cardiac conditions. And minerals like magnesium, calcium, and potassium are also very good.

Protecting a Healthy Heart

Q: I exercise and I try to eat right, and my doctor says my heart is healthy. I want to keep it that way. At 72, I see a lot of problems among my friends who haven't taken care of their hearts.

A: That's just great! To keep your heart healthy, consider taking some vitamin E. Don't take more than 800 milligrams per day. Some people I know use 1,000 to 1,200 milligrams per day, but nobody needs that much, and it's not safe. Eight hundred milligrams per day is my safety limit. If you are planning to have surgery, avoid vitamin E entirely. It inhibits platelet function and causes increased bleeding.

Q: Can I improve my diet?

A: Almost everybody can when the health of the heart is considered. What is your main source of protein?

Q: I don't eat much red meat. Mostly I eat poultry and some fish. I also eat a little cottage cheese, skim milk, and such.

A: That is an excellent diet! Try to work a little tofu into your diet. It's a nutritious soy protein that works against cholesterol. A few years ago it was hard to find tofu outside health-food stores, but now almost all regular grocery stores carry it. Lots of recipes are available, too.

When you're cooking, use plenty of onions and garlic; eat them raw, if you can. These improve your circulation and help prevent blood clots. They can lower both blood pressure and total cholesterol. Add lots of ginger to your diet because it improves circulation and digestion. Niacin is sometimes recommended for lowering cholesterol levels, but this should be taken only with your doctor's supervision. Too much niacin can cause liver damage and other problems.

RAYNAUD'S DISEASE

Q: My wife is 53, and she has Raynaud's disease. She's had her gallbladder removed and a hysterectomy, and she takes Premarin. She has low blood pressure, too, so our doctor has put her on Zestril.

I think the Zestril is a problem. If she doesn't take it, she gets migraines. If she does take the full dose, she becomes lethargic. She's reduced her dosage to about a quarter of what the doctor prescribed, and she feels better and doesn't get the headaches. I'm wondering if her Raynaud's disease anything to do with the headaches.

A: Something doesn't sound right. First of all, Raynaud's probably doesn't cause her headaches, because it's a microvascular disease of the extremities. The small blood vessels constrict—we don't know why—and cut off the blood supply from the affected area, usually the hands or feet. Does she smoke?

Q: Not for over twenty years. When we first discovered that she had Raynaud's disease thirty years ago, her fingers turned white. Now her hands turn black when she gets cold or she's under stress.
A: That's very typical of Raynaud's, and I think she needs a medication change. Today we use calcium channel blockers to treat this disease, not ACE inhibitors like Zestril.

Ginkgo biloba is very effective in improving circulation to the skin areas throughout the body. To strengthen your wife's circulation, add plenty of stimulants such as cayenne and ginger to her diet. Prickly ash may also help. Hawthorn whole-plant extracts are very good cardiovascular tonics; they increase the strength of the heart beat, the fluidity of the blood, and the strength of the blood vessels. A multivitamin with antioxidants will also be good for your wife. I'm not sure of the source of her headaches, but maybe they'll clear up when she gets her Raynaud's under control.

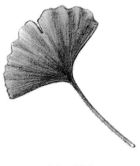

ginkgo biloba

CONGESTIVE HEART FAILURE

Imagine you have a sump pump in your basement and it's been raining a lot. The basement starts to fill with water. If the sump pump doesn't work to push the water out, you'll have a flood. With congestive heart failure, the pump—the heart—isn't working. The body retains salt and water, and the blood volume increases. Fluid pools in the lungs, causing labored breathing with even mild exertion, and eventually we see swelling in the feet and ankles.

Q: What causes this?
A: A damaged heart. Prolonged high blood pressure is a common cause of heart damage, as is heart attack, atherosclerosis, or heart-valve disease.

All result in a heart that can't pump efficiently.

When blood returns to the heart from the body, it first enters the top right chamber of the heart and then the bottom, flowing through the pulmonary artery into the lungs, where it is cleaned and picks up oxygen. The refreshed blood enters the pulmonary vein and flows into the top left chamber of the heart, then the bottom left chamber and the aorta, which carries it throughout the body.

Trouble occurs when the heart's pumping action can't remove all the fluid from the left lower chamber. The fluid backs up into the top part of the heart's left side and fluid from the blood collects in the lungs. The term for this condition is congestive heart failure.

Q: How can I prevent it?
A: Keep the heart healthy. Eat sensibly, exercise regularly, and control any conditions that may lead to heart problems, particularly diabetes, high blood pressure, and high cholesterol. And don't smoke!

One who already has congestive heart failure can use hawthorn extract to strengthen the walls of the heart's coronary arteries, lower blood pressure, and normalize heart beat. No side effects are known, and hawthorn can be used safely for long periods. And like all the cardio-vascular problems we've already discussed, diet, exercise, and stress relief are important to recovery.

ARTERIOSCLEROSIS AND ATHEROSCLEROSIS

Arteriosclerosis is the gradual thickening and stiffening of the arter-ial walls. Atherosclerosis refers to fatty deposits in the arteries. Either condition can lead to strokes, heart disease, and/or high blood pressure, but high blood pressure can also cause arteriosclerosis. It is also impli-cated in atherosclerosis because deposits are most likely to form in areas of the blood vessels that have been weakened by high blood pressure.

A heart attack occurs when the heart muscle is starved of oxygen and other nutrients because its blood supply is cut off, gradually or abruptly, by narrowed arteries or by a clot. The brain, on the other hand, is the site of strokes, which occur when an artery that supplies a portion of the brain is blocked. Without the flow of fresh blood, the brain tissue dies.

Q: *Is there any natural program that will reverse build-up of plaque in the arteries?*
A: Dr. Dean Ornish has done important work on reversing heart disease. In his book *Reversing Heart Disease,* he has shown that following a specific low-cholesterol diet, can be helpful. Otherwise, the only way to remove plaque from the arteries is by surgery or chelation therapy.

Chelation

Q: *I hate to see so many people dying or losing loved ones because they don't know about chelation therapy or are scared to try it.*
A: A chelating agent is a chemical that the body does not use but that has a slot, or hook, that fits an element we want to eliminate. The chelating agent catches the unwanted element, a molecule of toxic heavy metal, for instance, and carries it away for elimination.

For victims of heart disease, chelates attack calcium, the mineral that binds the plaque that forms in the large and medium-sized blood vessels.

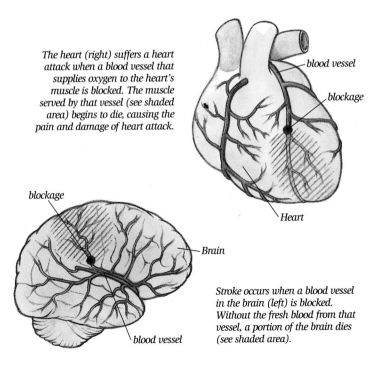

The heart (right) suffers a heart attack when a blood vessel that supplies oxygen to the heart's muscle is blocked. The muscle served by that vessel (see shaded area) begins to die, causing the pain and damage of heart attack.

blood vessel

blockage

Heart

blockage

Brain

blood vessel

Stroke occurs when a blood vessel in the brain (left) is blocked. Without the fresh blood from that vessel, a portion of the brain dies (see shaded area).

When the calcium is pulled out of the plaque, the entire structure falls apart and the artery is more open for blood flow.

Some chelates are administered by mouth, and these can be taken at home. They are safe, and they seem to be most useful in increasing circulation or restoring it in injured areas. Stronger chelates are administered through a vein, a process that requires a doctor's supervision. Several treatments are typically required to clear the blood vessels.

HEART RATE

Irregular Heartbeat

Q: I have heart flutters. When I lie down, my heart sometimes beats very rapidly for a half minute or so. I don't have high blood pressure or anything, so is this a problem?

A: Brief irregularities in the heartbeat are very common. They're caused by a little confusion in the electrical commands that regulate the heart's beating action. If your flutters are short and don't happen very often, they probably don't indicate anything serious.

An herb that helps regulate the heartbeat is motherwort, and you might consider using that to keep your heartbeat regular. How old are you?

Q: I'm 49.

A: Do you anticipate pregnancy, or are you pregnant now?

Q: Heavens, no! My children are all grown up and I'm a grandmother.

A: Good. Motherwort can stimulate uterine contractions, so pregnant women should avoid it. Otherwise, it's a very good remedy for heart palpitations. It calms the heart and also acts on an overactive thyroid, which often is the cause of fluttering heartbeats. Hawthorn is also an excellent herb for strengthening the heart.

If you notice a change in your heart flutters, be sure to let your doctor know about it right away. There are other kinds of arrhythmias that are quite worrisome and require treatment.

Q: Are there vitamin supplements that can help irregular heartbeat?

A: We've found that people with irregular heartbeat often have comparatively low levels of magnesium. Sometimes levels of phosphorus are low, too. Supplements of both minerals might be helpful to you.

Heart Rate and Alcohol

Q: My husband had a quintuple bypass operation four years ago. He is now 62, and his heart is back to about ninety-seven percent normal. He watches his diet fairly well—no sweets, large meal at noon, a light one in the evening—but he drinks rum and soda in the evening, maybe four or five glasses. He has always had a fast heart rate. He rides a bike five miles three or four times a week, doesn't take his blood pressure medication, but monitors his blood pressure regularly. I think he shouldn't have more than a drink or two per day. Am I right? He has just retired, and I would like him around a while to enjoy it.

A: He definitely should not have more than one or two drinks daily, no question about it. Four or five drinks are beyond anybody's standards.

Q: Is there anything he can do naturally to bring down his heart rate?
A: If your husband is biking as much as you say he is, he should not have a high heart rate. He should have his doctor check for a thyroid condition, heart-valve disease, or anemia. Any of these could be a problem.

Finally, are you sure he's not drinking more than you think he is? He should reduce his drinking, but it might be difficult. He may experience alcohol withdrawal and need medical support while he is withdrawing.

As for natural remedies, your husband would benefit from onions and garlic eaten raw or cooked. They thin the blood and ease the heart's job. You can buy garlic preparations that don't produce the smell or digestive upset that raw or cooked garlic sometimes does.

STRENGTHENING THE VEINS IN THE LEGS

Thrombophlebitis

Q: My dad is in his late sixties, and he seems to have a tendency to get blood clots in the legs. He's had several small ones, and I wonder if we can keep him from getting more.
A: What did your father's doctor say about the blood clots?

Q: He said not to worry about it, actually. He didn't give Dad any antibiotics or any instructions except to wear an elastic sock and to keep his legs elevated as much as possible. I do worry about it, however, and I would like to do whatever we can to prevent these.

A: It sounds like your father may have had some clotting in a superficial vein. What were his symptoms?

Q: *He had a sore red area on his lower leg. It felt like there was a cord under the skin, and the area was hot, so we thought it was an infection.*

A: I think your father had a superficial thrombophlebitis. It may occur from an injury to the leg, sitting or standing for long periods of time, or a sedentary lifestyle. We don't know precisely the cause, but it appears that there is some minor injury to the inside of the vein, and the body rushes platelets to the area, clogging the vein. These are painful, but they usually resolve in a couple of weeks. Moist heat often helps.

This does not mean that your father now has a serious concern, but he should be careful. He may be helped by taking garlic, to keep the blood flowing smoothly, and hawthorn extract or centella to strengthen the walls of the veins. Ginkgo biloba also increases circulation. Coenzyme Q10 and flaxseed oil, along with the minerals calcium and magnesium, may also benefit your father. Mild, no-impact exercise that gradually increases will stimulate his circulation. It's also a good idea to elevate the foot of his bed so that his veins drain well during the night.

Your father should promptly treat these clots when they occur, and he should work with his doctor to monitor the health of the deep veins in his legs. If he takes care of himself, he should stay healthy.

Venous Insufficiency

Q: *What can I do to relieve the swelling in my ankles and legs? I'm 71.*

A: There are various reasons for swelling in the legs, and one of the more common is venous insufficiency. The veins in the legs begin to swell and collect fluid and as a result you have some discomfort and swelling of the legs. Do you have any kind of heart problem?

Q: *No.*

A: Good. I'd suggest you elevate your feet as often as you can, and avoid salt because it will make you retain fluids. In addition, you may want to try hawthorn extract; it helps the cardiovascular system in many ways.

Eat lots of berries such as cherries, blueberries, and blackberries, or try extracts. Either form increases the integrity of the venous walls and strengthens the muscles of the veins.

We often see the situation that you describe prior to the development of varicose veins, so do watch this carefully. Also, be sure to mention the swelling to your doctor the next time you visit the office.

Varicose Veins

Q: What causes varicose veins?

A: Within each leg vein there is a valve that keeps the blood from rushing down to your feet when you are standing. The veins, you know, return blood to the heart, so they must push against gravity. If the valves within the veins become damaged or inefficient, or if the veins themselves become damaged, blood pools in the lower part of the veins.

Women suffer from varicose veins more often than men, especially during pregnancy or just after giving birth. People who spend many hours on their feet are also more inclined to get this condition; nurses and waiters, for instance, often have varicose veins.

There are a couple of things you can do about varicose veins. First, if you're overweight, lose the excess. Second, many insurance programs will pay for surgical support stockings fitted by your pharmacist, if your doctor prescribes them. The pressure of the stockings helps your veins resist pooling. Finally, elevate the feet so they are slightly above the level of the heart for fifteen to twenty minutes, three or four times a day. That helps to drain the legs. Walking will also help you because the action of the muscles encourages the veins to pump the blood back to the heart.

Q: Can I use any natural remedies to make my varicose veins go away?

A: I doubt that you can cure your varicose veins, but you can improve the situation. Extract of the herb *centella asiatica* can be very helpful when taken orally. It improves circulation, reduces hardening of the walls of the veins, and strengthens the connective tissue as well. Horse chestnut seed—yes, that's also known as Ohio buckeye—may also help, because it increases the ability of the vein's walls to contract and move the blood. Also try hawthorn berry extract, noted for its ability to strengthen the walls of the blood vessels. And eat plenty of cherries, blueberries,

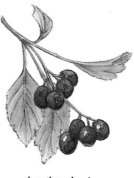
hawthorn berries

and blackberries.

Bromelain, the enzyme contained in pineapple, will help you, too. It helps prevent the hard, lumpy areas that often surround varicose veins. Some studies indicate that it also decreases the risk of blood clots.

The most important factor with your diet, however, is to be sure to include lots of fiber. Supplement with psyllium husk if necessary. Over the long term, include in your diet the foods that tone and strengthen the cardiovascular system: garlic, onions, ginger, and capsicum—that is, cayenne pepper.

Keep an eye on those varicose veins, too. If they're on the surface of your leg, they're ugly but less serious than if they are in the deep veins of the leg. If you feel more unwanted changes in your legs—heaviness, tiredness—let your doctor know. Deep varicose veins can cause serious blood clots that may move to the heart, lung, or brain.

BLOOD CLOTTING

Bruising

Q: My 80-year old mother-in-law is healthy and active, but if she bumps into something, even lightly, she gets gigantic bloody-looking bruises. What can we do to help her?
A: Is she on any medications?

Q: None. Not even aspirin. She very rarely takes any medication.
A: Bruising is the result of broken blood vessels beneath the skin. Once people are over 70, the superficial blood vessels are fragile. Both muscle and fat tissue break down, and capillaries that supply the skin with oxygen and nutrients become fewer. The connective tissue that gives skin its strength and resilience also deteriorates, so the skin is less pliable. Because oil and sweat glands are less active, the skin is dry and leathery. As if that's not enough, far fewer new skin cells are produced, and gravity's inevitable effects become clear. Bruising, slow healing, wrinkling and

various skin problems are very common among older folks.

Because bruising reflects a problem with the blood vessels, your mother-in-law should try ginkgo biloba to improve the blood supply to her skin. *Centella asiatica* is also a good possibility, for it improves the strength of the walls of the veins. Hawthorn will also help strengthen her circulation, and she might benefit from an antioxidant, too.

Q: Would calendula cream help? It's a natural cream that includes flowers, and it's supposed to help skin problems.
A: If your mother-in-law's skin is sore where she bumped it, calendula cream would be fine. It is very good for wounds, inflammations, and burns, but it doesn't really have any effect on the blood vessels that cause the bruises. But it won't hurt her, either.

Better for bruising would be a little rosemary essential oil diluted in a bland oil, perhaps almond oil. Rub it into the skin after the bruise has begun to heal, and it will actually help the body reabsorb the blood spilled under the skin. Be sure to dilute the rosemary oil, however, because it is quite strong and can cause skin irritation. Place a drop or two in a teaspoon of bland oil, perhaps canola or almond. Rub the diluted rosemary oil into the skin after the bruise has begun to heal.

Low Platelet Count
Q: I had my annual physical recently, and my doctor said my platelet count is down. What does that mean?
A: Platelets are components of the blood that serve to stop bleeding when there's a break in the skin. For instance, if you cut your finger, the platelets immediately come to the wound and form a plug by sticking to each other, preventing the blood from gushing out.

Aspirin inhibits platelet function by making the platelets less sticky, which is good if you have heart disease or a tendency toward clotting. But it's not so good if you cut yourself and can't stop the bleeding. Other anti-inflammatories have similar effects, and so does alcohol.

It's important to know your platelet count. If your count falls below one hundred, you're likely to have serious problems with bruising and bleeding.

Q: Is that related to anemia?

A: No. It has nothing to do with anemia. Your blood contains red blood cells, white blood cells, and platelets. Red blood cells carry oxygen to the cells, and if they're too low you are anemic. White blood cells fight infections, and platelets control bleeding. All three counts are reported on the complete blood count or CBC.

Q: So do hemophiliacs have low platelets?
A: No, hemophiliacs have a different kind of problem with blood clotting. There are twelve different clotting factors, and in hemophiliacs, Factor 8 is deficient. Blood clotting occurs in a step-by-step sequence, and in hemophiliacs a step is skipped, so the blood doesn't clot correctly.

Low platelet count does cause a condition called idiopathic thrombocytopenic purpura, or ITP. "Idiopathic" doesn't mean the doctor is an idiot and can't figure it out—it means nobody knows the specific cause of it. And the symptoms are often vague, too. Most frequently we discover it when doing blood work for something else, or sometimes we see some unusual bruising. But it's not terribly common, and the only treatment is prednisone.

Low White-Blood-Cell Count
Q: I'm 77 years old and have arthritis. I get my blood checked regularly because my white blood count goes way down. This has been happening for twenty years.
A: White blood cells (WBCs) fight infection. Lymphocytes and neutrophils are included in the WBC count because they have similar functions. Lymphocytes specialize in attacking viruses and neutrophils battle bacterias. There are other protective components as well, all of which are counted as white blood cells.

The normal WBC count is from four to eleven (depending on the laboratory where the tests are examined). Some people consistently have low WBC counts—three and a half, or even three—and they're still healthy.

If the WBC count drops below 2, it's a different story. Counts below 2 show a problem with infection or a susceptibility to infections because your immune system isn't functioning.

Quite honestly, if your WBC has been fluctuating for twenty years, you don't have leukemia or any other kind of cancerous condition. If you'd like, get a second opinion from a hematologist—a blood specialist—who may recommend a bone-marrow test. If your bone marrow has somehow been damaged, that would explain the fluctuation.

CARDIOVASCULAR DANGER SIGNS

Q: I'm 72. I want to know why these last few months my right arm has been going sleep. It also hurts.
A: When you say your arm is going to sleep, do you mean there's tingling and numbness?

Q: Yes.
A: Do any of your fingers bother you? Is your arm weak?

Q: My index finger and my ring finger hurt, but there's no weakness.
A: Please have your doctor check this out soon. I'm a little concerned because of your age, and this sounds a bit unusual. You definitely should tell your doctor about this, because it could be quite serious. Do it right away.

If you experience a heavy feeling or sensation of pressure or squeezing in the center of the chest for more than a few minutes, get to a hospital or call 911 promptly. Other warning signs of heart attack include light-headedness, fainting, sweating, or shortness of breath, but all these symptoms don't necessarily occur at once.

Stroke symptoms include sudden weakness or numbness of one side of the face, or of one arm or leg; double vision; sudden headache or dizziness; or unexplained falls. Strokes may be preceded by temporary attacks of numbness or partial paralysis that last only a few minutes or a few hours. These are often warnings of impending stroke, and require immediate medical attention.

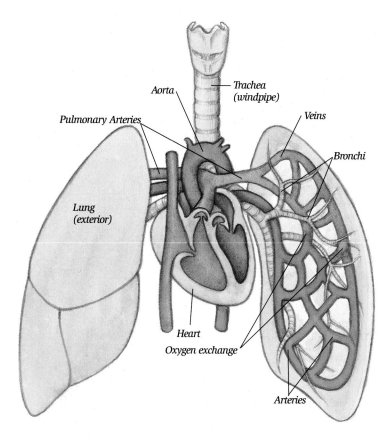

Aorta

Trachea
(windpipe)

Pulmonary Arteries

Veins

Bronchi

Lung
(exterior)

Heart

Oxygen exchange

Arteries

The Respiratory System

Respiratory Health

Breathing in, breathing out.

It seems so easy.

L ate in pregnancy, the lungs of the unborn infant lie shrunken and heavy in the chest cavity. They are firm, compacted, and dark red. At the moment of birth, the baby inhales her first air, and her lungs bloom. Swiftly they fill the chest cavity, becoming pink and spongy. As the baby's little heart beats and she breathes, her body begins circulating oxygen to every cell.

So begins the work of the lungs. We each take nearly eight million breaths per year, and with every one several essential events occur. First, we take in the oxygen that is necessary to life. The air is warmed (or cooled) to body temperature and purified before the oxygen enters the bloodstream. From the blood, the lungs take carbon dioxide and other waste gasses that the body doesn't need and exhales them. The lungs also produce an important chemical, angiotensin, that regulates blood pressure.

Dangers to the lungs are many. Some lung diseases, such as cystic fibrosis, are inherited. Smoking, of course, damages the lungs directly and severely. Avoiding smoking and pollution while keeping the body healthy and fit are the best approaches to healthy lungs.

THE COMMON COLD AND FLU

Hundreds of viruses can cause what we call colds and flu—infections of the respiratory tract—although, at any one time in a given region, only a few are active. While each virus is distinct, all can cause similar symptoms: headache, muscle aches and pains, cough, sore throat, fever, and runny nose. Flu sets in a bit more quickly than colds, but most folks don't know when they actually were infected. Generally, even health professionals call infections with less severe symptoms and discomfort "colds," and those that are more serious "flu." Without culturing the virus, it's impossible to identify which one or which type is causing the illness.

Contrary to common belief, getting chilly, perhaps by staying outside in cold weather without a jacket, will not make anyone catch a cold or flu. The likelihood of contracting the virus does go up, however, when you're overly tired, experiencing emotional distress, or fighting allergies that affect the nose and throat. For women, cold and flu viruses most frequently set in during the middle of the menstrual cycle.

Q: I have a friend who is a school teacher, and she's constantly exposed to children and all their colds. She catches cold, gets a sinus infection, and then bronchitis. What can she do?

A: People who are around children—teachers and child-care workers—are very likely to be exposed to respiratory viruses, of which there are many. As you can imagine, health professionals have the same problem. People come to see us specifically because they're coughing, sneezing, and aching all over. We're exposed to everything.

Preventing the spread of colds is the first line of defense. By maintaining a healthy diet, getting adequate exercise, and keeping your immune system in good condition, you decrease your chances of catching cold. A diet that includes cayenne pepper and garlic will help ward off colds, and both of these are available as tablets that are easy to take and don't upset the stomach.

Secondly, colds are spread primarily through person-to-person contact and by the aerosol droplets that hang in the air after someone sneezes. The virus can live outside the body for a time, so if a child with a cold handles a book and then gives it to another child, the virus goes along for the ride and may infect the second child. You can see why our schools and day-care centers often have micro-epidemics of these infections.

Everyone who works with children should make a habit of washing their hands thoroughly and frequently with soap and water. Children who are old enough should also be encouraged to do the same, especially when they've been in contact with other children who may be contagious. I believe that handwashing ought be part of every classroom's daily routine, and the teacher should participate as well as lead. Children should wash their hands when they come into the school, before every meal, before leaving for home, and certainly after using the restroom. We have essentially eliminated general health education from many schools, and if we can teach young children only one thing in this area, it should be this: Wash your hands often.

If your friend is regularly seeing a progression from cold to sinus infections to bronchitis, something is wrong. The symptoms of a cold normally resolve within five to seven days. Recurring secondary infections associated with her colds could indicate that her immune system is weak or that she has an ongoing problem in her respiratory tract. Either situation requires diagnosis, evaluation, and treatment. For that reason, she should discuss her situation with a physician.

Under typical circumstances, however, colds may be treated in a couple of ways. First, boost the immune system by taking echinacea at a cold's onset and continue it for ten days. Set it aside for a week and then, if you are not completely well, take it again for another ten days. So long as no fever is present, astragalus can be taken as needed; it also supports the immune system. Both vitamin C and zinc shorten the duration and the intensity of colds.

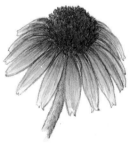

echinacea

Various symptoms of the common cold can be treated herbally, too. Goldenseal works as a cleanser and anti-inflammatory, although you should take it only a short time—ten days or so—and not at all if you are pregnant. Chickweed reduces the mucous buildup in the lungs; so do feverfew and fenugreek. A tea of horehound leaves soothes the throat and eases the coughing that often accompanies a cold.

I take a Chinese herb called andographis. It is available as a tablet or in tincture form. It is a fast-acting herb that is very safe. I've been taking it during flu season for two years, and during that time I've not caught either a cold nor flu.

How We Catch Colds

Q: As a massage therapist, I sometimes wonder if I can catch things from people I work on, or if they can get colds from me.

A: The main way colds are transmitted is by inhaling droplets from coughs or sneezes, and by using something that's been handled by someone with a cold. For instance, suppose someone with a cold uses an ordinary pencil. Then somebody else picks it up and uses it, and then touches his nose or eyes. The second person could possibly catch the virus. That's why having your own equipment and washing your hands is really important during flu season.

When Children Catch Cold

Q: My sister-in-law has a 5-year-old and sends him to preschool. He's there all day and catches a lot of colds. What can she do?

A: Prevention is the best strategy when dealing with colds. First, teach the boy to keep his hands out of his mouth and away from his eyes and to wash his hands often. The child also needs an excellent diet to keep his immune system healthy; during the cold season, extra garlic is good for him. I give my own children a pediatric dose of echinacea when they are coming down with a cold. They take it for seven to ten days, then stop for a week, then repeat another cycle of seven days if necessary.

My children also take acidophilus year round. Most bacterial or viral infections infect us by one of two routes: through the respiratory tract or through the gastrointestinal tract. A good bacterial coating of the intestinal wall prevents infectious agents from attaching, so they can't make you sick. For children, mix refrigerated, powdered acidophilus into juice or water. Children who go to day care can take it at home in the morning and evening.

Q: I have an infant, and now that she's going to day care she seems to be sick all the time. All the kids are. How can I prevent this? She's 4 months old.

A: Have you visited the day care center to find out if the workers are conscientious about washing their hands regularly? Also washing the hands of the little ones, too? It's important, especially during cold and flu season. If cleanliness is not a very high priority at the day care, perhaps you should look for one that is more cautious.

Before you give your baby anything, I suggest you consult a health-care professional who knows and understands both natural medicine and children. Usually it's okay to give the child pediatric or infant formulations designed to enhance the immune system or work in other ways against colds, but it's best to be sure. If you child does get sick, remember that antibiotics are effective only against bacterial infections, and colds are caused by viruses. Unless your child has a bacterial infection along with the cold, antibiotics should be avoided.

Reye's Syndrome

Q: I understand that if my child has a fever from a cold or flu, I shouldn't give him aspirin. Why is that?

A: It's because of a condition called Reye's syndrome. This is an inflammation of the brain and liver that attacks children who are recovering from a viral infection such as flu or chickenpox. Children who have had aspirin during the viral infection are up to thirty-five times more likely to get the syndrome.

Reye's sets in as the child is getting over the viral infection. Sudden vomiting and fever are followed by agitation, delirium, fatigue, and confusion. Without treatment, coma and death may follow. Although Reye's syndrome usually affects children, no one fighting a viral infection should take aspirin. White willow bark, an herb sometimes used for pain relief, contains an active ingredient very similar to aspirin, so don't use it, either. For colds and flu, use ibuprofen or acetaminophen.

Reye's syndrome is very serious and requires a physician's care, but with early diagnosis and prompt treatment, the prospects of recovery are excellent. After medical treatment, support recovery by using milk thistle to strengthen the liver and hawthorn to improve circulation and strengthen the heart. If the patient is anxious, a tea of chamomile or catnip is calming.

Flu Shots

Q: What do you think about flu shots? I got a flu shot last year and I still got some kind of flu. Do the shots really work?

A: Personally, I think everyone who works around a lot of other people should get a flu shot. Certainly anyone with a chronic illness such as heart disease or respiratory problems should have the flu shot, and elderly folks should, too. However, if one of my patients is reluctant, I don't try to talk him into it. Anyone with allergies to eggs should not have the flu shot, for the vaccine is prepared in a mixture that contains egg.

There are pluses and minuses to the vaccination, and everyone should make an informed decision for themselves. The flu shot protects only against specific viruses that epidemiologists believe will be predominant during that particular flu season; other viruses are unaffected. So the good thing about the flu shot is that if the experts have predicted correctly, and you've had your shot, you probably won't get that kind of flu. The bad thing is that you might get another kind of flu.

Garlic

Q: Does garlic help prevent colds?
A: Garlic contains allicin, which does protect against viral and bacterial infections. You can eat a few cloves daily or take enteric-coated capsules. Avoid garlic if you are taking blood thinners.

Protecting yourself or your children against colds and flu begins with frequent hand washing and the maintenance of a strong immune system. Echinacea is an excellent immune-system stimulant. Goldenseal reduces irritations of the mucous membranes.

COLD SORES

Q: Are there any herbal remedies for canker sores or cold sores? I get them all the time. They really hurt, and they look terrible.
A: Canker sores and cold sores are both caused by the herpes virus. Once you contract the virus—as nearly everyone has—it stays in the body for life. The virus hides from the immune system in nerve cells, and during times of stress, illness, or depressed immunity, it pops up again.

Q: Are canker sores different from cold sores?
A: No, they are both herpes infections.

Q: Is there any way to prevent them?
A: Balancing the intestinal flora helps stave off cold sores, and most people

can benefit from taking acidophilus to improve their resistance and immunity to these viral outbreaks. A strong immune system also defends against the virus, so eating an optimal diet that is low in refined sugars and flours, minimizing stress, and avoiding allergens are helpful. If you have regular outbreaks of cold sores, avoid chocolate, cashew nuts, hazel nuts, peanuts, chick peas, pecans, sesame seed, and walnuts. Eat plenty of halibut, shrimp, and salmon; chicken and turkey are good, too. Mung beans may also help.

When cold sores or canker sore do appear, the dietary supplement L-lysine prevents the herpes virus from growing. Take the L-lysine for one week, along with goldenseal. In addition, you can apply goldenseal extract directly to the cold sore; tea tree oil is effective, too. Licorice root is also helpful in suppressing the herpes virus, but don't take it if you have high blood pressure, and don't take it for more than a week. For pain, try a tea of gotu kola or catnip.

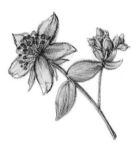

St. John's-wort

Q: Are there any creams that I can rub directly onto the cold or canker sores?
A: Yes, you can buy L-lysine in a cream. You can also find creams that contain zinc, which helps heal cold sores. If you can find St. John's-wort in a cream or ointment, it may be helpful because this herb also has relatively potent antiviral activity. If you take St. John's-wort internally, however, you may find that it causes you to sunburn quite easily.

SINUS CONGESTION

Q: My mother-in-law is in her mid-seventies and she suffers from sinus problems a lot. She can't seem to get relief from anything.
A: If her problems are related to allergies, she could try astragalus and echinacea. When you see her again, ask if she has a white coating on her tongue. If she does, she's likely to have stuffy sinuses and breathing passages. Does she live by a lake or by water?

Q: No, she doesn't.

A: Good. Folks who live near water more frequently have yeast problems and allergies to molds.

She may have some other kind of allergy that has become more severe with age. Allergies occur when the body attacks a common substance as though it were an infectious agent. Disease-fighting mechanisms roar into action, and that's why we see inflammation, localized swelling, fever, and general malaise in cases of severe allergy. Minor allergies have more moderate symptoms, but still cause discomfort.

The most common allergens are wheat, dairy, eggs, citrus, corn, and peanuts in any form. Your mother-in-law might benefit from eliminating these foods, first one and then another, from her diet to see if she improves. For instance, she should take care to eat nothing that contains eggs for one month. If her sinus congestion improves, there's a good chance she's allergic to eggs. The same process can be used to help identify other things that bother her sinuses, such as wool, cleaning supplies, or other troublesome elements in her environment.

Your mother-in-law could probably benefit from taking acidophilus to improve her digestion, and from an excellent diet that is high in fiber. If she's not allergic to ragweed, she should try echinacea and goldenseal to boost her immune system. Another strategy is to sniff a warm spoonful of goldenseal tea deeply into her nose; this bathes the sinuses with healing solution. If she has an acute, painful sinus attack, she could crush a good-sized piece of ginger root and apply it externally to her sinus areas. This will help relieve pain and promote drainage.

> *Allergies occur when ordinary substances activate the immune system.*

Q: I've never had allergy problems before, but now that we've moved to a new state I seem to be sniffling all the time. Over-the-counter sinus medications help, but I don't want to take them forever, and I don't want to take the scratch tests that the doctor gives to determine allergies, because they're expensive and often just tell you what you're NOT allergic to.

A: When do your allergies get worse or better? Have you noticed that certain foods or activities seem to bring on more symptoms?

Q: The more time I spend outside, the worse they get. If I stay in, they're not too bad, but when I work out in the yard or go walking, I notice a difference. When we go camping, they get worse.

A: It sounds like you might have an allergy to something in your new area's plant world. You may be able to build an immunity to local allergens by purchasing honey from a local source and using it in small quantities as you usually would—to sweeten tea, on toast, and so on. Be sure you get honey that bees make right in your area—honey from Illinois will not help develop immunity from allergens in Florida. Honey contains tiny amounts of pollen and other plant components that cause allergies, and by ingesting small amounts of the honey you may stimulate your own immunity to these factors.

Nasal Sprays

Q: I use over-the-counter nasal sprays when my hay fever acts up, but some of the products carry warnings against using them for more than three days. Is that because they're addictive, or because they'll eat away the inside of your nose?

A: Both. If you abuse these products they will destroy the tissue of your nose. I once had a patient who treated himself for an extended time for what turned out to be a very serious allergy, and his septum, the nose's little dividing wall, completely deteriorated. In addition, the body can develop a tolerance to the active ingredients of the spray, and some products do have addictive properties.

Following the directions on these products is essential; most indicate that the product should be used for only three days. More importantly, however, if you are troubled by a sinus or nasal problem for more than three days, you should see a doctor. It could be something more serious than a transient allergy.

ASTHMA

The symptoms of asthma range from alarming to terrifying to deadly. During an attack, overproduction of thick mucus in the lungs and spasms of the alveoli—the "leaves" at the very tips of the bronchial branches—interfere with breathing. Wheezing may be the only symptom in mild cases, but a range of symptoms characterizes severe cases.

Asthma arises from a variety of causes and individual conditions. Some asthmatics are affected by commonly inhaled allergens such as dust, mold, and animal danders, while others react to respiratory infections, exertion, inhaled chemical fumes, or even cold air—and some have multiple triggers to their attacks. Researchers have also identified some metabolic abnormalities and unusual personality components among asthmatics. The illness is most typically seen among children under the age of 10, and more often among boys than girls.

Q: My daughter, age 6, has been diagnosed with asthma, and we're very worried about taking care of her the right way. What can we do to help her?
A: Asthma is dangerous. Your doctor will help you learn what you need to know to take care of her, and you will have to talk with her school teacher and the school nurse about her condition and how she is being treated. The most important thing, though, is that you teach your daughter to care for herself. Even at 6 years old, there will be times when she is on her own and might have an attack. So she has to learn how to take care of her illness, and she's not too young to begin.

Every asthmatic must understand when to take action or get themselves to the emergency room. A simple device called a peak-flow meter can be used at home to monitor peak flow or lung capacity, and every asthmatic should be using one and know what his or her normal peak flow. When the peak flow falls below normal, the patient needs to know exactly how to respond, either by taking a treatment, informing the doctor, or getting to the emergency room.

Q: Do you know of any natural remedies that will help her? We want to do everything we can.
A: Do you know what causes her asthma?

Q: No, but I think the doctor has taken some tests to try to answer that.
A: When you get that information, it will be easier to figure out how to treat her. Asthma is usually brought on by food allergies, extremely sensitive airways, or an unusual chemical reaction in the body. Until you have a good idea of the cause of her asthma, however, you might try a

vegan diet, one that eliminates any products from animals. That means no cheese, no eggs, no milk or yogurt, as well as no meat or fish. Also, eliminate chlorine from her diet with a water filter.

She should eat lots of fruit and nuts, especially blackberries, blueberries, and strawberries. Plums and pears are good, but not apples or citrus fruits. Nuts, whole grains, and all the vegetables except soybeans and green peas will help her, and she should have potatoes in limited amounts. Some children with asthma who use this diet improve within four months, and after a year most are improved.

Supplement her diet with vitamins B_6 and B_{12}, and give her plenty of vitamin C, too. Asthma patients often have low levels of these vitamins in their bodies, and they improve when they get the supplements. Magnesium is helpful, too, because it eases tension in the air passages.

When you have a better idea about what triggers your little girl's asthma, work with her doctor, and do your own research, to design a complete treatment program for her. Most cases of asthma are very manageable.

Q: My little boy has always been a little bit nervous, and now he has asthma. Our doctor says his attacks are mild, but the boy gets frightened and upset by them, and that seems to make his attacks worse. Is that possible?

A: You may be quite right about your son. Dr. Stewart Hochron, a lung specialist and a good friend of mine, has done excellent work on personality and asthma. He's found that certain personality characteristics create a predisposition to asthma or incline an asthmatic to more frequent or more severe attacks. Many asthmatics are very anxious, uptight, or nervous, and they secrete an excess of hormones that constrict the nasal passages and blood vessels and promote bronchial spasms.

Q: What can we do about it? He's always been like that, I don't know how to make him less nervous.

A: Find an instructor for your son who will help him with relaxation and biofeedback techniques. Dr. Hochran's study found that meditation and relaxation helped asthmatics control the catecholamine release and reduce their bronchial spasms. Biofeedback was successful in helping asthmatics slow their heart rate and breathing. Using these techniques may help your

Biofeedback and relaxation techniques can reduce asthmatic spasms.

son gain control over his illness. He really needs to learn to care for himself properly, and this can be an important part of it.

Q: What herbs would be safe to use for my asthma? It comes from allergies, so some triggers might be related to herbs.

A: If you want to use herbs for your condition, make sure they are not related to the plants that trigger your asthma. For instance, echinacea, a popular herb for stimulating the immune response, is a member of the aster family. If you are allergic to ragweed, one of its relatives, echinacea can cause problems for you. You can get plant information from an herbalist, a good herbal reference book, or perhaps from the botany specialists associated with your county extension service.

Q: What herbs should I look into, then? Which are good for asthma, assuming I'm not allergic to them?

A: You could try licorice root, which is quite good for various respiratory problems—bronchitis, sore throats, congestion—but be sure it is deglycerrhizinated if you also have high blood pressure. Licorice is both antiallergic and anti-inflammatory, so it helps asthma. Ephedra, which is an active ingredient in many cold medicines, should not be taken by anyone with high blood pressure; otherwise, however, it reduces mucous secretions and improves respiratory tract function. Slippery elm bark, an herb used by Native Americans, soothes irritated passages and relieves coughing when taken as a tea.

The diuretic qualities of saw palmetto berries are valuable if the asthma includes excess fluid in the bronchial passages. It's also an effective overall cleansing agent. Vitamins B_6 and B_{12}, along with magnesium, potassium, and water, are also important. Remember that asthmatics need plenty of clean water to lubricate the secretions and keep them as loose as possible.

STREP THROAT

Q: My daughter gets strep throat once or twice a year. I take her to the doctor right away, and he prescribes antibiotics for her, and she gets well. But six months or a year later, we repeat the whole process. I think she's getting too many antibiotics, and I'd like to treat her strep with herbs instead.

A: I understand your concern about this, because it's true that antibiotics have been over-used in some situations. However, I always caution my patients that antibiotics are the definitive treatment for strep throat. Herbs and vitamins and supplements are not fast enough, or powerful enough, to protect your daughter from this dangerous infection. When she has completed her antibiotics, however, get her on acidophilus to prevent yeast from overtaking her intestinal flora or from multiplying elsewhere in her body. Use goldenseal to boost her immune system, and teas of mallow, raspberry leaf, or lungwort to soothe the soreness of her throat. Get plenty of garlic into her system, too, as it has antibiotic properties and will fight the streptococcus bacteria that cause the infection.

Strep is making a comeback. The World Health Organization has identified strep as one of the four most virulent diseases in the world. Left untreated, it can destroy the kidneys by causing glomerular nephritis. Pediatricians always screen for strep, but adults can get it, too. An acquaintance of mine ignored his strep throat and ended up needing a kidney transplant. Please take your daughter's infections very seriously.

BRONCHITIS

Q: I've gotten bronchitis three times this last year. Each time, I get a cold first, then bronchitis. Antibiotics clear it up, but I'd like to get rid of it for good. I do smoke, but only about half a pack a day.

A: Don't smoke. Every time you smoke a cigarette, your bronchial tubes and lungs become irritated, and they secrete extra protective mucus. The mucus then begins to plug the bronchial tubes, closing the airways. You have shortness of breath, you provide a prime opportunity for infection, and you stress the heart. When you smoke, the blood receives too little oxygen, and the heart must pump harder and faster to circulate the inadequate blood. Over the long run, your bronchitis can become chronic. It can also lead to pneumonia. At half a pack a day, you're a candidate for serious lung problems.

Q: What do I do?

A: First, throw out the cigarettes. You should also heal your respiratory tract. Use an excellent diet low in refined sugars and flours and high in leafy vegetables, whole grains, and lean meats. Eat no dairy products or eggs; these stimulate the formation of mucus. Boost your immune system with goldenseal, taken for one week. Vitamins A, C, E, and B complex and garlic, a natural antibiotic, will also protect against infection. Drink lots of good water; that will keep the bronchial mucus thin and in motion, helping to unclog the bronchial tubes.

Quitting Smoking

Q: I'd really like to quit smoking, but I just can't. I can get through the first five days or so, but then I feel so jittery and nervous that I've got to pick up a cigarette. Are there any herbs or vitamins that can help me?

A: That's just great to hear. What motivated you to quit?

Q: I have a terrible cough, especially when I get up in the morning. To tell the truth, my little girl asked me to quit smoking so I could be her mommy for a long time. They get taught in school that people who smoke don't live very long, and that really bothered her.

A: I applaud you for your effort, and please give your daughter an extra hug for me. She has saved your life.

Quitting smoking is tough. Some say that tobacco is more addictive than cocaine. Nicotine addiction seems to combine physical and psychological dependence, so quitting requires a broad strategy for success. Overcoming your smoking habits is the key to quitting for good. First, remove all smoking materials and smoking reminders from your home: every ashtray, every match and lighter, every cigarette pack. Then make your home a strict no-smoking area for everyone. If you eat a meal in a restaurant, seat yourself in the no-smoking section. If you regularly light up a cigarette when you dial the phone, move the phone away from your comfort area; if necessary, just don't use the phone for a while. If you like to sit down when you smoke, do things that require standing up. And clean your home thoroughly, especially draperies and carpets, to remove that smoky smell.

During this time, try various forms of ginger to encourage sweating;

ginger helps remove nicotine from your system. When you feel nervous, use a calming herbal tea like chamomile, or take valerian. Vitamins C, B, B_{12}, and E will help your body heal the damage from smoking. Grapeseed extract as an additional antioxidant is also good. Slippery elm bark tea helps loosen mucus in the lungs and bronchial tracts.

When you feel the urge to smoke, get up and do something else: take a walk, scrub the kitchen floor, dig in the garden. Physical activities help to break the smoking habit. In three months or so, your shortness of breath will improve, your sinuses will clear up, your cardiovascular system will be more efficient, and your energy level will be up. In short, you will feel a lot better.

Q: I'm worried about gaining too much weight, though. I don't want to get fat.

A: If you eat a healthy diet that includes very little meat or dairy products but lots of vegetables, whole-grain products, and plenty of fiber, you won't have to worry much about gaining weight. And look at it this way: If you do gain weight, you can lose it. But if you lose your lungs, you can't replace them. Good luck!

TUBERCULOSIS

Q: I'm aware that when people live in crowded or unsanitary conditions—for instance in prisons or inner cities—tuberculosis has become a danger again. Plus they say the new TB is resistant to antibiotics. Can alternative medicines help?

Quitting smoking is tough, but herbs can help.

A: Tuberculosis—even the suspicion of it—requires immediate attention from a physician. Our generation has never seen tuberculosis. From the old movies, we think that people with tuberculosis grow pale and thin and die in a sweet, graceful manner. It's not that way at all. Tuberculosis can affect any organ of the body, causing ulcerations of the skin, ruptured aorta, severe arthritis, and female infertility.

Only a few years ago, we thought tuberculosis was a thing of the past; the tubercle bacillus was nearly eliminated. Now, with the incidence of HIV and AIDS, it has returned with a vengeance. In fact, when we diagnose tuberculosis today, we immediately suspect a compromised immune system.

The disease spreads when an infected person coughs, creating a cloud of droplets in the air, and another person inhales the droplets some time during the next several hours. Tuberculosis is not as easy to catch as a cold, because people normally fight the infection off. Those with suppressed immunity, however, are quite vulnerable, especially if they live as part of a group or in an institution of some kind.

The issue of antibiotics resistance complicates treatment considerably. The drugs traditionally used against tuberculosis are no longer effective against these super tuberculosis strains, so for a full-blown case of TB we may use three or four different antibiotics. Like the older antibiotics, the full course must be taken according to instructions, not just until the patient feels better. That's a problem in populations that have little stability in their lives, such as the homeless and the drug-addicted.

Unfortunately, tuberculosis threatens to present a serious public health problem again. People in the health-care field should have yearly tests to make sure they haven't been exposed. Children should have patch tests done as part of their routine immunizations. Clearly, a strong immune system is the best defense against tuberculosis, especially if you are in a high-risk population or associate with someone who is.

WHEN YOU MUST SEE A DOCTOR

Q: I've had a cough for a while and I wonder if there's anything I can take for it.
A: Tell me about your cough. How long have you had it? Do you cough up any sputum?

Q: I've had it for a couple of months, I guess. I thought it was a cold because I've had some fever off and on with it, sometimes it gets pretty high. And lately I've been coughing up a little blood with the sputum.
A: Have you seen your doctor about this?

Q: No, I don't have a doctor. We just moved here a few months ago.
A: You need to find a doctor right away. The cough you have described

could indicate a serious problem, and you need a thorough examination, tests, and a solid diagnosis. Then, when you know what the problem is, you and your doctor can discuss possible treatments.

Any time a persistent cough is accompanied by a high fever, either constant or intermittent, you should see a doctor. Coughing up blood under any circumstances is cause for alarm. Other danger signs involving the lungs are breathlessness or shortness of breath, chest pain, sweats or chills, and bluish skin or cyanosis.

These symptoms may indicate lung problems, or they can indicate problems of other systems. Shortness of breath, for instance, may indicate pneumonia or lung abscess, or perhaps heart failure. Cyanosis may indicate that the lungs are not operating efficiently, or it may indicate that the blood vessels are not operating correctly. Your doctor must evaluate your symptoms and your health history to determine the likely cause of the problems.

When serious symptoms appear, you must contact your physician. Trying to diagnose and treat yourself can waste valuable time that may be needed to treat a serious condition. I advocate the patient's taking responsibility for good health, and part of the patient's job is contacting the physician when experiencing worrisome symptoms. Waiting too long to take this step can allow your condition to worsen and delay your recovery.

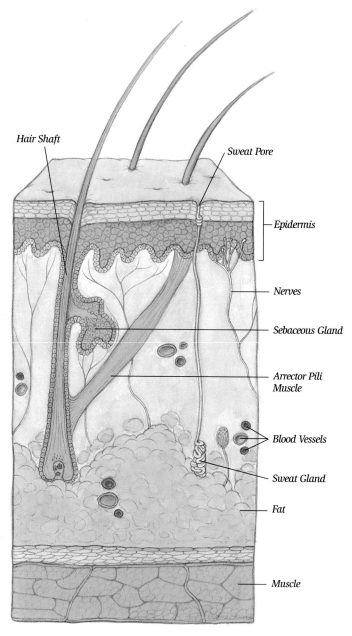

Hair Shaft

Sweat Pore

Epidermis

Nerves

Sebaceous Gland

Arrector Pili
Muscle

Blood Vessels

Sweat Gland

Fat

Muscle

The Skin (Cross-Section)

SKIN PROBLEMS AND ALLERGIES

A healthy diet creates healthy skin.

The skin is the mirror of the body's internal condition. As the body's largest organ, the skin protects it from many harmful environmental substances. By perspiring, the skin eliminates waste and regulates body temperature. Healthy skin is smooth, flexible, clear of blemishes, and neither pale nor reddish looking.

Skin that is irritated by external or internal imbalances responds in several ways. Rashes or blemishes, dryness and flaking, discolorations, and thickening are just a few of the symptoms skin displays when it needs attention. When skin irritation does occur, look for an underlying cause or imbalance. For example, the condition known as intertrigo, an outbreak where two skin surfaces rub together, such as the groin, between the toes, or beneath heavy breasts, may result from an overgrowth of candida. The moisture, friction, warmth, and sweat retention in those places encourage the growth of bacteria and yeast, and the skin becomes soft, reddened, and susceptible to more serious infections. When the body's internal problem with candida is addressed and healed, the intertrigo may clear up. Skin problems such as dermatitis, eczema, and other rashes often result from contact with external irritants, although the source can be dietary problems, too.

The word "dermatitis" means "inflammation of the skin" and does not indicate a specific kind of outbreak or a certain cause. When dermatitis breaks out, it's important for the patient to think about possible sources of irritation. For instance, when did the outbreak occur? Were you busy with a new activity that day, or the days before that, or were you in a new environment? Suppose the problem began the week you started spring gardening; you had been handling numerous plants from the nursery and digging in the soil. You may have been exposed to nursery chemicals or soil elements that irritated your skin. Identifying the source and correcting it is a major step toward healing the skin problem. In this case, wear gloves to protect your skin and soothe redness and itching by applying vitamin E to the rash.

Daily nutrition, however, plays the most important role in maintaining good skin health. Think about this: If you eat a poor meal of over-processed, greasy food that's been held on steam tables rather than freshly cooked, you are going to feel crummy the next day. If you continue such poor nourishment, your skin will soon tell the tale, although you may not realize why.

On the other hand, a healthy diet will be reflected in that beautiful "healthy glow" we all admire. If you have any skin problems, immediately eliminate from your diet all wheat, oats, rye, barley, and dairy products for six weeks; many people see an improvement in their skin from this step alone. Make sure your diet contains plenty of fiber, too, which will help keep the colon clean and healthy. Avoid fats, sugar, and processed foods, and completely eliminate alcohol and caffeine. If you do all this, you will have quite a healthy diet; to give your skin a boost, supplement with a vitamin B complex, vitamin E, and zinc.

PSORIASIS

Chronic and unpredictable, psoriasis afflicts one in every one hundred people. Itchy, scaly, round or oval patches develop on the skin, sometimes after a skin injury or a streptococcal infection like a sore throat, but more likely without cause. Heredity has a bearing on one's risk of psoriasis, but the condition is not contagious. Many patients report long-lasting remissions.

Q: My mom has had psoriasis for a number of years, and she says that the medicine she's using now is working better than any other, but it's

very expensive. It's a cream she rubs on the psoriasis.
A: Is it a topical steroid?

Q: Yes, and I wish we could do something preventive instead. Her medicine is very strong, and I'm worried about her using it for a long time.
A: Topical steroids, the preparations applied to the skin, are not absorbed into the system and are safe for most people. On the other hand, steroids taken internally, like prednisone, suppress the adrenal glands when they are used over long periods. Pregnant women should avoid internal steroids. These medications can cause all kinds of serious side effects such as cataracts; they accelerate osteoporosis, because steroids rob the bones of calcium; and they can cause other systemic problems. If your mom is using her medication properly and it's helping her, I wouldn't worry about it.

As to prevention, psoriasis treatment varies a great deal from one person to another. Some improve if they add citrus fruits to their diets, but others get worse with the same remedy. Nearly everyone with psoriasis improves, however, when they eat better food. So take a look at your mom's diet. She should probably cut down on refined flour—pastas, for instance, and white bread—and replace these carbohydrates with rice, quinoa, and other grains. In addition, reduce or eliminate dairy products, fats, and sugar.

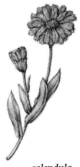

calendula

When your mom has a flare-up of her psoriasis, it would help to gently brush the scales from the sore and apply an extract of goldenseal, making sure that the extract contains no alcohol. She can also simmer a bit of lavender oil in water just hot enough to create steam, and hold the psoriasis sore over the steam. Both these herbs stimulate healing. A cream containing calendula will also soothe the outbreak.

ACNE

Acne, the bane of adolescents, afflicts four out of five teenagers. Diet is the primary cause, and perhaps heredity, and possibly hormones.

Blackheads, pimples, and cysts typically flare up during hormonal swings when androgens, male sex hormones produced in the bodies of both males and females, stimulate the growth and production of the sebaceous glands. These glands, growing larger and secreting more sebum—the oil that lubricates the skin—can become clogged and sometimes infected. Despite the marketplace's determination to convince acne sufferers that one preparation or another will completely prevent or eliminate acne, most bouts usually last only a week or two, although some cases persist for years, or for life.

While hormonal development and imbalances are typically blamed for acne outbreaks, I believe that acne is more closely related to diet and digestion. During the teenage years, young people ignore their parents' directives about nutrition, and they eat more meals away from home: snack foods, fast food, candy, and the like. Typical young people have diets high in salt, fats, and refined ingredients, and they drink soda, not water. In short, few pay any attention to nutrition. Soon the acne crops up, and the hormones are blamed, but it's really the diet of young people that is causing the skin problems.

Q: My son is 15, and he has serious acne. My other kids had occasional breakouts, but this boy gets deeply infected pimples almost like boils, and they appear not only on his cheeks and forehead but now on his neck and shoulders, too.

A: Your boy's sebaceous glands are larger and more numerous in these places. That's why you see the acne there. How does he feel about his condition?

Q: He's really upset about it. It's so bad that he stays home as much as he can to avoid having anyone his age see him. He hangs around with only a couple of other boys—which I don't understand because he's very bright and funny, at least when he's relaxed.

A: Acne is awful for young people. They get it just when they're feeling most insecure about themselves, their future, their attractiveness to the opposite sex—and a bad case of acne can leave emotional scars as well as physical ones. He needs prompt help to heal his acne.

First, make sure that your son has a good diet and eats plenty of green vegetables. Teenagers, given the choice, would probably subsist on french fries and chocolate, but emphasize to him that he must practice good nutrition to overcome the acne. Further, remove the refined flour, sugar, food additives, and all animal and hydrogenated fats from his diet, and put in plenty of fiber and complex carbohydrates. Acne often clears up after a month or two with these simple changes.

> *A bad case of acne can leave emotional as well as physical scars.*

Acidophilus, as far as I'm concerned, could help your son more than anything. By balancing intestinal flora with helpful acidophilus bacteria, toxins are eliminated more easily through the intestine rather than through the skin. Thus, the skin's job becomes easier, and it heals faster.

Your son ought take supplements of beta-carotene, vitamin C, and zinc. Echinacea is good to boost the immune system, but don't take it for more than ten days. Finally, calendula is a soothing, antibacterial herb, and a calendula tea applied directly to the acne—particularly when a pustule has opened and drained—is helpful. Aloe vera gel, one of my favorites, is also soothing and healing. He should keep his skin clean, of course, but not overly dry from too much washing.

Finally, if your son is otherwise healthy, encourage him to get plenty of exercise. Working up a sweat helps the skin perform its function of eliminating toxins, and it's good for him in general.

If none of this is effective, and your son continues to get large unsightly acne, you should take him to a dermatologist. Certainly take into consideration his ability to be patient about his condition; if he becomes overly anxious about it, don't delay that visit to the doctor.

Q: My daughter is 14, and she breaks out just before her period. She gets one or two glaring, inflamed spots on her face, usually in the same places. I think that's pretty normal, but she's so embarrassed and upset she wants to stay home from school. Can we be doing anything to prevent these monthly spots?
A: Focus on your daughter's diet, making sure that she gets good nutrition and enough fiber; a clean colon is essential to clear skin. Particularly be certain that she is getting enough zinc, which helps prevent outbreaks.

Of course she should be keeping her skin clean.

Because her acne appears to be associated with her monthly cycle, your daughter may benefit from drinking a mild tea containing dong quai the week before and the week of her period. This herb helps normalize the hormonal swings that can contribute to acne problems. When she breaks out, applying a little tea-tree oil to the lesion will help eliminate infection; a bit of lavender oil in a hot bath is both soothing and healing. A non-oily aloe or calendula cream to keep her skin soft will help, too.

Finally, do what you can to keep your daughter free of stress during these times. When she's feeling upset, chamomile tea, which is very calming, may help her relax and find relief from whatever is troubling her. There's nothing like a little tea and sympathy from Mom!

ROSACEA

Q: I'm 32, and I'm in good health, but I've developed acne. I can't believe it! I didn't have much of an acne problem when I was a kid, but now that I am old enough to have kids of my own, my face is red and sore-looking, I'm breaking out, and it hurts quite a bit sometimes.

A: It sounds like you don't have simple acne; I think it's rosacea, a chronic flushing and eruption of the facial skin that's pretty common among middle-aged and older adults. Women have it more often, but men get the more severe cases. We're not sure what causes it, but it might be a bacterial infection, B-vitamin deficiency, or perhaps a digestive imbalance. Menopausal flushing or alcoholism could also be factors, and sometimes we see rosacea in families. Rosacea can be fairly minor, or it can be so serious as to cause scarring, particularly on the cheeks and nose.

Q: Can I treat it? Can I get rid of it?

A: Rosacea, like psoriasis, is a very individual condition. What helps one person doesn't necessarily help another. We do know that drinking alcohol or hot liquids, being in the sun, exposure to extremes of temperature, and eating spicy foods can aggravate rosacea, so stay away from those.

You must be on a healthy diet that encourages clear skin. Also, consider supplementing your diet with evening primrose oil, which has healing properties, and vitamin A. In addition, vitamin B complex with a high proportion of B_{12} is helpful.

Herbs that you ought to try are alfalfa, milk thistle, and burdock, all taken internally. The alfalfa helps in healing, and the milk thistle supports the liver in cleansing the blood. Burdock root, taken internally, cleans the blood and also improves skin tone. Also, apply calendula cream to nourish the skin.

Q: You didn't say how I can get rid of rosacea.
A: Rosacea is chronic; that is, it persists over a long period of time. Treatments help, but you may always have it. Don't ignore it and do keep treating it. Untreated rosacea can cause unsightly scarring.

SHINGLES

Q: My uncle got shingles in his ear, apparently as the result of a small cut. How could this happen?
A: Shingles is a very painful rash that actually begins with chickenpox, the *varicella zoster* virus. Toward the end of the child's bout with chickenpox, the virus migrates along the major nerves to the spinal area and lies dormant. Later, often decades later, the virus reactivates; in this form, it's called *herpes zoster,* or shingles.

We see shingles most often when the patient has experienced a chronic illness, chemotherapy, emotional stress, or another situation that has suppressed or overtaxed the immune system. Unfortunately, elderly people are the most likely to experience these problems, and thus the most likely to develop shingles.

Shingles begins with flu-like symptoms, along with burning and itching at the site where the shingles will develop. Most people don't recognize the symptoms as the start of shingles. When the serious pain and the rash start, however, most people go promptly to the doctor for treatment.

The rash of shingles—red bubbles and lesions—don't cross the midline of the body. If the shingles appears on the right side of your body, for instance, you will not see it on the left side. The virus affects only the area served by the nerve in which it lay dormant, so it can't appear on both left and right sides. This inflammation of the nerves creates extreme pain—shingles makes people feel just miserable.

Although shingles is fairly common, don't take a casual attitude about it. Shingles on the face is a medical emergency. If you have it on the tip of the nose or anywhere around the eyes, you need hospitalization with intravenous antiviral therapy. If the virus involves the facial nerve and gets into the eye, you can go blind without warning. Shingles can be very serious, even fatal, for those with impaired or suppressed immune systems. Shingles confined to the ears does not constitute an emergency, but you still should be very cautious.

Because there is no cure for shingles, treatment concentrates on shortening and minimizing the pain. Zovirax and Acyclovir are antiviral medications for shingles, and both work to neutralize the virus. Echinacea helps boost the immune system; it should be taken for ten days, but no longer. St. John's-wort, skullcap, and oatstraw tinctures, mixed together in equal parts and taken four times daily, a teaspoon at a time, are calming and relieve the pain and itching of the shingles rash. Some shingles rashes heal more quickly when exposed to sunlight for short periods daily, say about fifteen minutes. Finally, vitamins E and C will help the healing process.

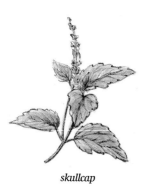

skullcap

Q: *Grandma has shingles. Does that mean she can't visit her grandchildren because they could catch the chickenpox from her?*
A: Absolutely. If your grandmother's lesions are open, she shouldn't be around anyone who has not had chickenpox. When the pustules, or fluid-filled bubbles, are open, they are full of virus and Grandma is contagious. When the pustules dry up, which usually takes a week or ten days, Grandma can visit again.

PEELING FINGERTIPS

Q: *I have very dry skin at the end of my fingers and around my cuticles. The skin peels and doesn't heal.*
A: Bag balm is very good for this condition. There are several brands on the market; it's a creamy preparation that was originally used to heal

irritations on the udders of cows. And it works! Quilters love it because their hands get dry from working with fabric so much; you can often buy bag balm at quilting shops and other fabric stores.

You can also mix acidophilus powder with sterile water to make a paste and apply it to those rough spots. Fresh aloe is also very good for promoting healing.

ENVIRONMENTAL ALLERGIES

Q: I've been putting up wallpaper. My husband has been helping me some, but he's a heart patient and had an adverse reaction to something, maybe the wallpaper adhesive. The label warns about a fungicide that reduces mold on the paper. His upper lip swelled and turned wrong side out and his throat got real red.

But I'm also thinking maybe he developed an intolerance to his medications. When we consulted his doctor, he immediately changed my husband's Lotensin to Tenoretic.
A: First, how long has your husband taken the Lotensin?

Q: About a year and a half.
A: Your husband's reaction is probably related to what you were doing in the house. Reactions to most medications usually happen soon after taking the medication—certainly within a day or two. The exception is antibiotics. An allergy to antibiotics can occur at any time.

Your husband probably had a reaction to something in the new materials in the house. It happens all the time—the amount of chemicals and finishes and sprays used in manufacturing household items is unbelievable. Many are toxic and can become airborne.

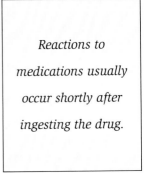

Reactions to medications usually occur shortly after ingesting the drug.

When you place these new things in your house, especially during winter, the chemicals become concentrated. Many people react with mild symptoms such as headache, nausea, or fatigue and probably don't associate the discomfort with the new living-room set.

I recommend that when you are making improvements to your home, or moving into a new house or a new work environment, you use an ozonator or an air purifier to draw all the chemical junk out of the space. What with new carpets, new floors, new fabrics, even airborne dust and debris from remodeling, amount of contaminants can be astonishing. Nobody needs that kind of stress on the immune system, so I recommend this protection.

Q: Is there any way to know for sure whether my husband has environmental allergies?
A: The best way to determine if you have environmental allergies is to get out of the environment for a time, then return to it. If the symptoms disappear, or are noticeably relieved when you are away, but flare up again when you return to the environment, there is strong evidence to suspect allergy.

I've worked as a physician for an industrial firm, and more than once people have come to me complaining that they feel fine all weekend, but Monday when they come to work they start feeling a little off, and by Friday they are feeling quite ill. Now, people joke about their jobs making them sick, but for some it's true. When this happens over and over again—healthy weekends, sick work weeks—allergy is a very strong possibility. The source of the allergy can be one factor or several of many, many factors that are present in the work place, and, unfortunately, some workers simply have to get new jobs because they are unable to live with the symptoms of allergy.

CONTACT DERMATITIS

Q: What is contact dermatitis? I have these red, swollen patches on my hands, and I can't think of anything I've been doing differently.
A: Contact dermatitis is an allergic skin reaction to a particular substance. To treat it, whatever causes the outbreak must be removed. Do you regularly put your hands in strong substances, chemicals of any kind?

Q: Well, yes, I work as a hairdresser, but I've been doing that for years. If I were allergic to any of the perm solutions or hair products that we use, I think I would have known it long ago.

A: I know this is hard to believe, but you can become allergic to anything at any time. Adults can develop allergies the same as children, even when they have been exposed to the allergic substance regularly. Do you put your hands in any other chemicals or unusual substances?

> *Adults can develop allergic reactions just as children can.*

Q: No. I like to refinish furniture in the summer, but since it's cold now I haven't done that for several months. I wear rubber gloves when I'm handling those chemicals, like the directions say, and I've never had any trouble.

A: Try wearing rubber gloves while you are using hair products, too, and see if your dermatitis clears up. The only way to get rid of the rash is to protect the skin from coming into contact with what causes it.

When your rash flares up, mix a little goldenseal root powder with some vitamin E oil and add a bit of honey to make a paste. Apply that to the rash to ease the itchiness and help in healing.

Q: Could it be something else? I'd hate to be allergic to stuff I have to use every day.

A: There are many sensitizers—substances that can provoke allergic reactions—used in the manufacture of our shoes and clothing. These include tannins, antioxidants, and dyes. Cosmetics ingredients also cause allergies in many people, and the ingredients are always changing. Many people are allergic to nickel or other metals, especially when alloyed; pierced ears or other pierced body parts can become very painful if this allergy develops. And of course the innumerable industrial compounds that we're exposed to create reactions as well.

Q: I hope I'm not one of those people who has to leave a job because of allergies. I love my work.

A: You might try a cruise ship.

Q: I don't understand.

A: One of my patients told me about a hairdresser she knew. Her friend developed terrible contact dermatitis from perm chemicals, and nothing helped. She was forced to go on disability and was quite discouraged.

Then she learned that cruise ships almost always have beauty salons, and that very few people ask for permanents there. She applied, got the job, and now sails around the world doing the work she loves and seeing beautiful places, too. And she's healthy. So her skin allergy turned out very well for her.

WARTS

Q: My little boy has a couple of warts on his fingers. I know the warts can be cut off or burned off, but is there something that would not be so traumatic for him? He's just 6 and a little bit afraid of doctors as it is. I don't want him to have a frightening experience if we can avoid it.

A: One thing you can do is nothing—most warts disappear on their own in a year or so. Warts are caused by a virus, and there is some evidence that they appear during or after a time when the immune system is stressed. They disappear as the immune system strengthens. For that reason, in addition to making sure that your boy has an excellent diet, I advise a supplement with vitamins B complex and C. These will encourage normal skin-cell reproduction and support the immune system. Garlic, which has strong antiviral action, can be helpful, too. Peel a clove of garlic and cut it in half; rub the cut side of the clove on the wart several times a day. Don't mash the garlic and bind it to the wart area, though, as it could harm the skin around the wart.

If the warts are stubborn, try a paste of castor oil and baking powder. Mix it up at the boy's bedtime and coat the wart well, then put a soft bandage on the area overnight. During the day, remove the bandage and paste. Some people have reported success with applying Vitamin E oil to the wart, too. Whatever treatment you use, continue it for at least six weeks.

BOILS

Q: What exactly is a boil? I think my husband has one. He got a sore, red area on the side of his neck, and suddenly this awful sore popped up. It looks like it has a core, but I can't tell for sure. He says it hurts a lot.

A: It could be a boil. If it is, be careful because boils are caused by a bacteria called *Staphylococcus aureus,* which is quite contagious. Be particularly careful when the boil comes to a head and drains, because the pus carries the bacteria. I've seen patients who have gotten more boils from the original one in this way, and members of their families have become infected, too. And yes, as your husband says, boils can be very painful.

A boil begins deep in an irritated hair follicle, usually on a part of the body that is covered with clothing and receives a lot of friction, such as the breasts, neck, buttocks, or under the arms.

Q: That makes sense. This sore is right where my husband's collar rubs against his neck.
A: That's very typical. You say that the sore seems to have a core, but you're not sure?

Q: Yes. There's a tiny white spot in the center but the sore isn't pointed. It doesn't look like it's ready to drain.
A: The last thing you should do with a boil is try to open it yourself, either by sticking a needle in it or pinching it or anything of that nature. If you do, you're almost certain to spread the infection. Keep the skin very clean by washing the area several times a day and applying an antiseptic. Otherwise, don't disturb the area of the boil at all.

You can, however, ease the pain and help the boil along in its progress by applying moist heat. Simply soak a clean cloth in very warm water and apply it to the sore until the cloth cools. Then repeat the procedure, using a clean cloth each time to prevent the spread of infection. This treatment, carried out for twenty minutes three or four times a day, will encourage the boil to drain spontaneously.

When the boil does drain, wash the area thoroughly with antibacterial soap and very warm water. Wash your hands thoroughly as well, and any linens or clothing that may have come in contact with the bacteria. Keep the area covered.

Goldenseal can also effectively treat these infections. It is excellent against microbes, and it promotes rapid healing, too. Make a thick paste

> *Boils are very contagious and must be treated carefully.*

of goldenseal root powder and a little water and coat the boil with it. Apply the paste several times a day, and keep the sore area covered. You could try over-the-counter antibiotic ointments, too.

Q: I don't want my husband to keep getting boils. Is there any way to protect him?
A: Good thinking! When we deal with the underlying causes of health problems, the benefits for healing, energy, and overall well-being are often more than we expected.

Remove from your husband's diet all the white flour, sugar, refined foods of any type, alcohol, and simple carbohydrates like candy. Supplement his diet with the antioxidant and healing vitamins A, E, and C; they boost the immune system. Zinc has proven effective in cases of recurring boils.

Q: What about the boil he has now?
A: If you don't see healing by two days after the boil has drained, consult a physician promptly. These infections can spread into adjacent tissue and become generalized; worse, they can get into the blood stream. That's a very serious situation.

You should also seek a physician's aid if more boils develop despite the diet change. Sometimes boils indicate an underlying illness such as diabetes or kidney problems. While such cases are rare, your husband should have a good checkup if the boils recur.

RINGWORM

Q: My daughter came home from summer camp with ringworm. She has it in her hair. I can't believe the place was so dirty that my girl came home with worms! Can I get rid of them?
A: First, ringworm isn't a worm at all, but a fungus infection of the skin's surface. And don't blame the camp. Ringworm is extremely contagious and spreads quickly on contact. So your daughter could have gotten it from another child, or from patting a dog that wandered through the camp.

You can treat ringworm quite effectively with natural remedies. Tea tree oil, an antifungal, attacks ringworm. Put eight or ten drops of the oil into a quart of warm water and dab the mixture onto the ringworm three or four times a day. See that your daughter is taking acidophilus; an imbalance of intestinal flora makes her more susceptible to fungus infections such as this. And make sure she eats plenty of garlic—she may prefer the deodorized capsules—because garlic is active against fungus.

Because ringworm is so contagious, your daughter's clothing and bed linens must be scrupulously clean. Everything that touches her skin must be washed after each use. Isolate her hairbrushes, combs, and so on from those of other members of the family, and wash them in hot soap and water after every use. When the ringworm is healed, replace all those things for the sake of safety.

Keep an eye on Fido and Puff, too. Household pets can get ringworm, so if you see any patchy hair loss or unusual skin appearance on your pets, take them to the veterinarian right away.

SUNBURN

Q: My family really enjoys outside activities, especially in the summer, but we all sunburn easily. Is there some kind of natural protection against sunburn? My daughters want to have dark suntans, but first they burn a couple of times.

A: The best treatment for sunburn it to avoid it, and your children must be taught to take sunburn seriously. Not only is sunburn painful and unsightly, it also causes long-term damage to the skin. Wrinkles, brown spots, and leathery texture to the skin are only the beginning; a history of sunburn substantially increases the chances of skin cancer.

When the skin is overexposed to sun, the ultraviolet rays create burns identical to one that might occur if you scalded your hand with hot coffee. Most cases of sunburn are first-degree burns that are red, painful, and warm to the touch; peeling often occurs. Severe sunburn, a second-degree burn, produces more redness, swelling, and fluid-filled blisters. Very severe cases include nausea, delirium, fever, and chills.

Fair-skinned people, especially blondes or redheads, are most susceptible to painful sunburn, but folks with darker complexions burn, too. Folks who work or play outside receive much more exposure to the sun than others and should take special precautions against skin damage.

Certain medications, and even herbs, may increase your susceptibility to sunburn. Taking tetracyclines and other pharmaceuticals may increase photosensitivity; always ask your pharmacist about this if you are taking a prescription medication. Various perfumes and colognes, especially those containing bergamot compounds, and some soaps applied to the skin increase the chances of sunburn. St. John's-wort, an herb often recommended for its calming qualities, also increases sensitivity to sunlight.

The best way to prevent sunburn is to wear clothing that protects the skin and to use sunblock that has a sun-protection factor (SPF) of 15 or higher. I know of no herb that will prevent sunburn. Wearing protective clothing such as wide-brimmed hats, long-sleeved shirts, and long pants will also help the skin.

Because the rays of the sun are strongest in the summer months and between the hours of 10 A.M. and 3 P.M., play in the sun when it is less harsh. And don't be deceived by a cool, cloudy day. The ultraviolet rays pass easily through light clouds, fog, or a foot of clear water, and cause serious sunburn. Snow, sand, and bright sky also compound bright sunlight by reflecting the sun's rays.

If sunburn does occur, herbs are very helpful in relieving pain and helping the healing. Aloe vera, preferably squeezed directly from the fresh plant, soothes the pain and helps heal the skin. It can be applied every hour. If you use a commercial aloe product, make sure that it contains no alcohol, oil, or wax that will sting or coat the skin. A strong tea of chamomile, cooled and applied to a clean, soft cloth which is laid over the sunburn, will also decrease the pain. Tea of gotu kola or comfrey has the same effect.

Infection can easily follow sunburn. Apply a cream containing calendula to the sunburned skin; this herb has antiseptic properties. Also, eat plenty of garlic, which is antimicrobial as well.

If your daughters continue to insist on deep suntans, consider enlisting the help of your physician. A serious discussion of the risks of sunburn and seeing medical pictures of some of the results of sun damage to the skin may convince your daughters that suntans aren't worth the risk.

SKIN DANGER SIGNS

There are a number of skin conditions that require the attention of a physician, preferably a dermatologist. These conditions should not be treated at home, nor should a visit to the doctor's office be delayed.

Scabies, an infection of the itch mite *Sarcoptes scabiei*, causes terrible itching as the female mites tunnel into the skin's surface to deposit eggs. The irritated skin is likely to become infected.

Any change in the skin of a diabetic is cause for a quick trip to the doctor, too. Diabetes deadens the nerves in the extremities, so wounds, rashes, or other skin abnormalities can go unnoticed and become seriously infected. In fact, in patients over the age of 40, gangrene is fifty to seventy times more frequent among diabetics than among nondiabetics.

Finally, any moles or other irregularities on the skin should be regularly inspected. Normally harmless, such spots can develop into real trouble. The American Cancer Society has devised the ABCD system to help people check their moles. If a mole or other skin growth shows any of the following signs, you should see a doctor, preferably a dermatologist, immediately:

A: Asymmetry, or an irregular shape. If you neutrally divided the spot in half, the pieces are not approximately the same size or shape.

B: Border irregularity. The border of the spot is ragged, blurred, or notched rather than smooth.

C: Color. The spot is not a single color, but includes darker, lighter, redish, or blue/black areas.

D: Diameter. The spot exceeds the diameter of a pencil eraser. While spots that are smaller can be troublesome, larger spots are more likely to need treatment.

You should also see a doctor right away if there is any other sudden change in a mole, or any rapid growth. When it comes to the ABCD of your skin, you can't be too cautious.

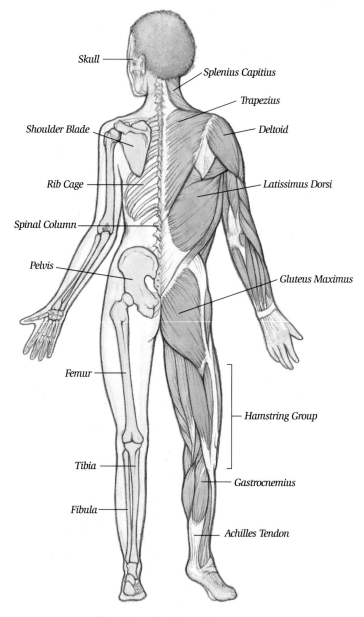

Skull

Splenius Capitius

Trapezius

Shoulder Blade

Deltoid

Rib Cage

Latissimus Dorsi

Spinal Column

Pelvis

Gluteus Maximus

Femur

Hamstring Group

Tibia

Gastrocnemius

Fibula

Achilles Tendon

The Musculoskeletal System

MUSCULAR AND SKELETAL SYSTEM

Structure and proportion, movement and strength—these depend on healthy muscles and bones.

The bones and muscles provide the body with form, strength, and the ability to move. While we usually think nothing of walking across the street, waving hello to a neighbor, or sewing a button on a shirt, each of these movements requires a lot of cooperation from the bones and muscles. Only when our normal daily activities are disrupted by soreness, swelling, or aching do we recognize the pleasure of a pain-free, responsive system of muscles and bones.

Over six hundred muscles are situated throughout our bodies, and all are devoted to providing movement. The striated muscles are those we use in our daily activities. If we wish to pick up a pencil, nerve impulses from the brain activate the striated muscles of the shoulder, arm, and hand, and perhaps others. Many other muscles function without our awareness. Smooth muscles perform numerous tasks in the body's organs; moving food along in the intestines is one example. A third type of muscle, cardiac muscle, exists only in the heart.

The bones give the body its individual structure and proportion, and particularly the unique form of the face. The skull and rib cage protect delicate organs from possible trauma, and the pelvis is the unborn child's first cradle. Blood is produced in the bone marrow. The bones themselves are constantly regenerating; in a healthy person, as old bone tissue wears out, strong new bone grows in its place.

Tendons and ligaments join muscle to bone and bone to bone.

Without this connective tissue, movement would be impossible. Other structures support the movement of the muscles and joints; the articular cartilage, for instance, cushions bones in joints, allowing them to move smoothly and painlessly. The synovial membrane surrounds the cartilage and parts of the bone, creating a nourishing liquid environment that preserves the joints' integrity. When cartilage or membranes deteriorate, pain follows.

BACK PROBLEMS

Back problems arise from many sources: old or new injuries, disks that no longer cushion the vertebrae as they should, habitually poor posture. Back pain might come from damaged muscles, a problem with the skeletal structure, irritation of the nerves, or a combination of these or other factors. Consequently, back problems are sometimes quite difficult to diagnose and treat.

Q: I have quite a lot of pain in my back. It hurts in the center of my back, just about where the lower ribs attach. A heating pad helps some, but then it hurts again the next day.
A: What does your doctor say about your back?

Q: Nothing, yet. I haven't been. I hate to go and then be told to do what I've already been doing, like put heat on it.
A: The first thing you should do is go to your doctor for a diagnosis. Back pain is caused by numerous ailments. What you feel may not be a back problem at all, and your doctor can rule out other serious conditions whose symptoms include back pain. And if your back *is* the problem, the doctor will prescribe correct treatment. Not all back problems are treated the same.

Among the conditions your doctor should rule out are colon cancer and prostate cancer. For women, ovarian and uterine cancer can cause back pain. Kidney stones, gallbladder problems, and osteoporosis may also show up as back pain.

Here's a story about how dangerous undiagnosed back pain can be. I had a patient who came to the office with a back problem and occasional abdominal pain. He had no history of hernia or trauma, heavy lifting, or back injury, but his back was causing him a lot of discomfort.

With my stethoscope on his belly, I heard a murmur that indicated an abdominal aortic aneurysm, a bulge in the blood vessel that occurs when the wall of the vessel is weakened. The aorta runs from the heart down through the front of the abdomen. At about the belly button, it divides to send blood to each leg and the lower abdominal area. Arterial plaque and aneurysms are quite common at the division point, especially among men who smoke and have high blood pressure, diabetes, and high cholesterol.

The rupture of an aortic aneurysm is followed by sudden, severe pain, rapid blood loss, and perhaps shock and death; it is a very dangerous condition. This particular patient had immediate and successful surgery to repair his aneurysms. He also had no more back pain.

Recovering from Back Pain

Q: Is it necessary to stay in bed every time you hurt your back? My husband thinks that's the best treatment, but I wonder.

A: Your husband is a little behind the times. A study in several medical journals reports that people with back problems or minor back injuries recovered much more quickly with physical therapy than did a similar

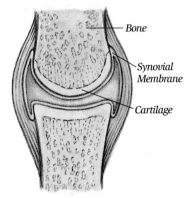

In a healthy joint, above, the bone ends are cushioned by cartilage and synovial fluid.

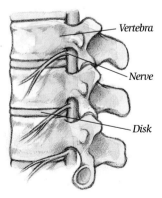

In the healthy spinal column, above, the vertebrae encase the spinal cord, the disks cushion one vertebra from another, and the nerves are not pinched or restricted.

group assigned to bed rest. People with mild back strain do much better when they resume their normal activities because movement and exercise promote circulation, reduce inflammation, and ease muscle tension.

Some alternative therapies are very helpful in relieving back pain. Acupuncture can relieve pain and reduce inflammation and spasm. Massage is also very effective in helping to resolve back problems. If you are interested in these alternatives, seek a qualified health practitioner who has extensive experience and training.

Q: I think I've hurt my lower back. My two-year-old had a tantrum and when I bent to pick her up, she threw herself backwards. I caught her before she hit her head, but my back was hurting by that evening, and it hasn't stopped aching. Is something like that enough to cause several days of back pain?
A: Back injuries aren't always dramatic. Sometimes even a slight injury results in a very painful problem. The structure or the architecture of the back may be involved. The source of the problem may be a muscle or one of the disks that separates and cushions the vertebrae. An injured muscle requires far different treatment than a disk problem, so you need an exact diagnosis from your physician.

If the problem turns out to be a simple muscle strain, you can treat it by applying ice packs to the painful area for the first forty-eight hours, then heat afterwards. Since you've had this pain for several days, I'd recommend a good hot bath daily, and perhaps a heating pad at other times when the pain is bothersome.

Once your pain is gone, you can strengthen your abdominal muscles by doing "crunches," which are now recommended by exercise experts to replace sit-ups. Lie on your back with your knees bent and place your hands behind your head. Using the abdominal muscles, lift the shoulder blades off the floor, hold momentarily, and lower the shoulder blades slowly to the floor again. Also, give your back a good stretch. While on your hands and knees, arch your back as high as you can, rest, and repeat. As with any other exercise, start slowly with a few repetitions and work up. The abdominal muscles are essential in supporting the back and preventing back injuries.

SCIATICA

Q: What's the best treatment for sciatica?

A: Sciatica is radiating pain through the buttock and down the leg. The pain may be intense and occur with low back pain or alone. The most common cause of sciatica is a herniated or slipped disk in the lower back that presses on the sciatic nerve and irritates adjacent muscles.

A herniated disk occurs when the cartilage disk between two vertebrae moves out of place. Healthy disks work as shock absorbers; when you stand or jump, the bones of your spinal column do not rub together because the donut-shaped disk lies between them. An injured disk, however, slips out of place between the vertebrae; it often protrudes between the bones. In this position, it can press and irritate the nerves that join the spinal cord; it can also cause local muscle inflammation and soreness. When the sciatic nerve is irritated, it is quite painful. Typical treatment is bed rest, pain killers, and muscle relaxants; at times, surgery is recommended.

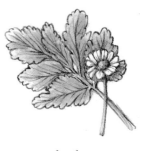

feverfew

To ease the pain, you could try the herb white willow bark, and take feverfew against inflammation. You also need the minerals calcium, magnesium, and potassium to strengthen your bones. Rosemary leaves are good against pain, inflammation, and spasm. B vitamins are helpful because they work to heal the irritated nerves.

OSTEOPOROSIS

Osteoporosis is a progressive disease that causes the bones to become thin and brittle. It is most prevalent among women, who begin to lose bone mass at about the age of 35. Bone loss accelerates around the age of 50, when estrogen levels decline and menopause begins. The affected bones appear normal in shape and size, but their density is diminished. The weakened bones are subject to fracture, most frequently at the wrists, hips, and lower spine.

Q: When I went to visit my mom, she said she has a little osteoporosis.

That worries me.

A: That's understandable. Osteoporosis is painful and dangerous for older women, and they should guard against it. Is your mother past menopause? Is she taking estrogen?

Q: *Yes, she's taking estrogen. I don't know the dosage. And she's taking calcium and a multivitamin.*

A: That's good. Hormone replacement therapy is quite effective in slowing the rate of osteoporosis, but there is some evidence that after a few years it loses its effectiveness in protecting the bones. Does your mother exercise?

Q: *Yes, she participates in a water-exercise class where she does walking and stretching in a warm pool.*

A: Good! You might encourage your mother to take up regular walking, and maybe do some very light weight-training, too, if possible. Exercise that puts healthy stress on the bones alerts the body to deposit more calcium there. The body will build up the bones at any age if it gets the right signals.

Remember the weight-training craze some years ago that recommended using kitchen items like cans of tomatoes in place of dumbbells? That's a good way for your mother to begin a weight-training program. She may not want to hang out at the gym to do her weight-training, so this way she can work out home by using a cans of tuna as weights and progress to lifting cans of grapefruit juice. A book about beginning weight training will help her devise a simple routine.

Q: *The reason Mom told me about her osteoporosis is I said I thought she looked shorter. Is that possible?*

A: The weakness of your mother's bones is allowing gradual collapse of her vertebrae, the bones that protect the spinal column. This makes her look shorter because she is stooped. The spinal column is the nerve center of the body. Terrific pain and paralyzing damage can occur when the spinal column collapses because one or more vertebrae give way. Keeping her bones healthy ought to be a high priority for your mother.

Healthy bones ought to be a high priority for you, too. Because your mother has osteoporosis, your chances of developing it later in life increase. If you take this advice to heart and protect your bones, your golden years can be healthy and happy ones. I certainly hope you do this.

Calcium Supplements for Osteoporosis

Q: My wife says I ought to be taking calcium to prevent osteoporosis. I say it's a female disease, and I don't think I need the pills.

A: You should listen to the wife on this one. Eighty percent of people with osteoporosis are women, but the other twenty percent are, of course, men. And very few men are aware they ought to be taking extra calcium. You also should be sure to get enough magnesium and vitamin D, which help transport calcium into the bones.

Calcium is important to prevent osteoporosis in both men and women. The recommended dosage for postmenopausal women is 1,500 milligrams per day. For premenopausal women, starting around the age of 20, it is 1,000 to 1,200 milligrams per day. Pregnant and breast-feeding women need 1,200 to 1,500 milligrams per day. Men over 60 should take 1,200 to 1,500 milligrams of calcium a day. Take it along with a magnesium supplement, which helps the body use the calcium, and vitamins A, E, and D to slow the aging process.

There are various forms of calcium. I don't recommend calcium carbonate, which is easiest to find. Calcium citrate, calcium lactate, and calcium gluconate are easier for your body to use. I particularly like the liquid supplements because they are much more easily assimilated.

Very few men are aware that they need calcium supplements.

WHEN YOU MUST SEE A DOCTOR FOR BACK PAIN

Several back problems require prompt care from a physician. If your back pain lasts for more than three days, or is getting worse on the third day, you should visit your doctor. Other serious symptoms are pain radiating into your leg, unexplained weight loss along with back pain, and pain on one side of the back along with nausea and fever.

If you are injured and have numbness or difficulty moving any limb, do not attempt to move. Instead wait for someone to call an emergency vehicle for you. You may have injured your spinal cord, and moving can spoil your chances for recovery.

HEEL SPURS AND PLANTAR FASCIITIS

Q: I have a heel spur in my right foot. Also plantar fasciitis. Is there anything I can do about this? My doctor gave me something for pain, but I don't want to take it indefinitely.
A: A spur is a calcium growth that protrudes from the surface of a bone. Depending on where it grows, it can be very uncomfortable. Plantar fasciitis is an inflammation of the fascia in the bottom of the foot. The fascia is the smooth covering of the muscles, tendons, and ligaments.

When you sleep, your entire body relaxes and the feet assume their normal, semiflexed position. When you awake and get out of bed, the fascia stretch along with the tendons and ligaments as the foot opens and flattens. If the fascia must stretch over an abnormal growth like a bone spur, the process can be very painful. When you awaken in the morning, sit on the side of your bed and stretch the bottom part of the foot by gently pulling your toes up and toward you. Do this three or four times through-out the day. Maybe at your afternoon work break you could take your shoes off and have a good stretch.

Here's another stretching exercise: Stand at arm's length from a wall, and place your hands on the wall straight out from the shoulder. Your feet should be together with your toes pointed at the wall. Then bend your elbows until your nose touches the wall, or until it's as close as you can get. Straighten your elbows to return to your beginning position. In short, do a push-up against the wall. That will stretch the calf muscle, the Achilles tendon, and the fascia of the feet, because they're all connected in your leg and feet.

EXERCISE INJURIES AND THE BACK

Q: I try to exercise regularly but I get muscle strains.
A: First, let's define exercise. The definition of aerobic exercise is a sustained heart rate for a sustained period of time. You can calculate your top heart rate by subtracting your age from 220. Always check with your

physician regarding your target heart rate. Most people should exercise enough to reach a heart rate of sixty or seventy percent of their top rate, and then work on sustaining the rate for increasing periods of time. Exercise twenty to thirty minutes a day, three to five times a week.

But actual exercise isn't the cause of most exercise injuries. The number one reason people get hurt during exercise is that they don't warm up prior to beginning the exercise. Instead, they jump right in. Their cold, stiff muscles are vulnerable to injury. The stress on the heart, which has been asked to speed up suddenly, can also bring on a cardiac crisis in some cases.

To avoid injuries during exercise, include a proper warm-up and cooldown in your routine. A good warm-up is five to ten minutes of the exercise you plan to do; if you bicycle, for instance, ride slowly for the first five to ten minutes, then speed up. At the end of your exercise, again ride slowly to allow your breathing and heart rate to return to near normal. Then stretch your major muscle groups; a ten-second stretch of each group—without bouncing, which can cause microtears and pain—will decrease the amount of muscle soreness you feel later.

Take care during exercise to replenish the fluids you lose through perspiration. Many of us were taught years ago to avoid water during exercise, but now we know that we should drink plenty. If the exercise is vigorous or sustained, you may also need to replace electrolytes—magnesium, calcium, and potassium. Special sports drinks provide these minerals along with fluid.

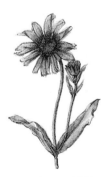

arnica montana

What can you do if you do get hurt? For sprains and strains, apply a cold pack immediately. Leave it on for ten minutes, then off for ten minutes. You may reapply in the same manner three or four times a day. Arnica montana is available in a cream for injuries like muscle strains and bruises; it also comes in homeopathic preparations. Glucosamine sulfate helps to lubricate the joints. Shark and bovine cartilage pills can be used for inflammation. Anything that opens up the blood vessels, such as garlic or hawthorn, also speeds healing.

Ligaments, tendons, and cartilage, which are the tissues damaged in sprains, tend to heal slowly because they don't have much blood flow. Muscular injuries heal more quickly due to their increased blood supply. If you get muscular cramps or leg cramps at night, be sure you're getting enough magnesium, potassium and calcium along with plenty of fluids.

ARTHRITIS

Arthritis forces millions of people annually to alter their activity because of pain in the joints, and it is the leading cause of disability in the United States. The term "arthritis" simply means "inflammation of the joints," and over one hundred different conditions that attack both the structure and function of the joints fit under this broad umbrella term. Swelling, redness, pain, stiffness, and even deformity of the body's moveable joints are symptoms of arthritis.

Arthritis has afflicted people of all ages throughout time. Its ravages are as apparent on the mummies of ancient Egyptians as in our own aching knees today. The cause of it was unknown in ancient Egypt, and the disease is only a little better understood today. A fundamental defect in the immune system is almost surely one cause, but genetic predisposition, biochemical disorders, and endocrine imbalances may also be involved. We also know that metabolic disorders, infection, trauma, and perhaps psychological factors may influence arthritis.

Arthritis attacks the linings of the joints and sometimes the bones themselves. A healthy joint is composed of at least two bones that are cushioned from one another by smooth, rubbery cartilage covered by a thin membrane, the synovial membrane, which secretes a thick fluid and surrounds all the structures of the joint. All the structures are vulnerable to arthritis.

Rheumatoid arthritis, the most common type, is the result of the immune system mistaking the synovial membrane for "nonself" and attempting to destroy it; the resulting inflammation and scar tissue damage other joint structures. On the other hand, osteoarthritis typically reflects the wear and tear of living, and results from degenerated cartilage. The bone ends, normally smooth, become rough, and sometimes bony spurs develop that further aggravate the joints. Arthritis in almost all its forms has a gradual onset. Remissions are common and sometimes long-lasting.

Q: Can arthritis be helped with herbs?

A: Natural medicine definitely plays a role in managing arthritis. Over time, patients experience both effective therapy and diminished side effects when they work with natural remedies. Because there is no cure for arthritis, patients must develop their own long-term care of the joints and management of the illness.

First, there may be a connection between diet and arthritis. Some research indicates that the nightshade family of vegetables—tomatoes, potatoes, eggplant, and peppers—contains a substance that picks up calcium and deposits it randomly throughout the body. If the calcium is deposited in joints that are already inflamed and painful, they will get worse. Other research indicates that those whose diets are high in refined flours and sugars suffer more arthritis than those who have a healthier diet. In my practice, I ask my arthritic patients to eliminate all nightshade vegetables, including nicotine, from their diets for one month. Then gradually add one type per week and monitor the progress of the arthritis. If the addition increases the arthritis symptoms, take it out again. Some have very good results relieving their arthritis pain by eliminating one or more of these vegetables. Eliminating white flour and sugar may bring relief.

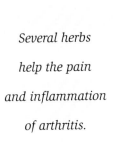

Several herbs help the pain and inflammation of arthritis.

Reducing the inflammation of arthritis decreases the pain, and several natural remedies fight inflammation. Feverfew is a good anti-inflammatory, and fresh (not canned or frozen) pineapple contains an enzyme that helps in this way, too. Glucosamine sulfate and shark and bovine cartilage have anti-inflammatory properties. The glucosamine sulfate has the added benefit of increasing lubrication to the joints. Bilberry stimulates the microcirculation around the joints and promotes healing.

Arthritis and Bleeding Ulcers

Q: What is the connection between a bleeding ulcer and rheumatoid arthritis? Several people I know have both.

A: I can't say for sure about your friends, but we usually see this combination in patients who have been taking large doses of anti-inflammatories for their rheumatoid arthritis, usually over a long period of time. Eventually, these medications damage the lining of the stomach, creating the ulcer. Aspirin is particularly bad; the nonsteroidal anti-inflammatories like ibuprofen are good pain relievers, but they too are very hard on the stomach. If you have kidney disease, diabetes, or high blood pressure, be very careful with over-the-counter anti-inflammatories.

People with ulcers should consider licorice, which is wonderful for healing the ulcer and soothing the entire digestive system. If you have high blood pressure, be sure you get the form called deglycerrhizinated licorice, because ordinary medicinal licorice can increase blood pressure.

Polymyalgia Rheumatica

Q: My doctor says I have polymyalgia rheumatica. What can I take for it? I have some other problems as well, including severe fatigue. I'm 55.
A: First of all, do you exercise?

Q: I can't do much because of the fatigue. I'm just so tired all the time.
A: Polymyalgia rheumatica causes severe pain and stiffness in muscles, but not permanent weakness or deterioration. It is often accompanied by fever, depression, and weight loss. We just don't know what causes it. One of the best things you can do is start an exercise program. Most cases of this illness respond rapidly to treatment with prednisone, a steroid. It's not my favorite medicine because of the side effects, but most patients do need it acutely, but the dose ought to be tapered off as soon as possible. A few do need to stay on the medication for longer periods. How's your diet?

Q: I've been trying to eat a lot of fiber, but I don't eat much fruit. I probably eat too much wheat and sweets.
A: There is nothing worse for you than candy, cookies, and sweets. I would be willing to bet that if you stop the sugar completely and begin taking acidophilus, you will start to feel better. Your concentration will improve, and your pain will be less. It won't happen overnight—it might take a good month—but the long-term effects are wonderful. I've had several rheumatic patients who have improved by changing their diets, taking acidophilus, and exercising.

Ankylosing Spondylitis

Q: I have ankylosing spondylitis. I'd like to know what kind of herbs or vitamins you recommend for this condition.

A: Ankylosing spondylitis, like many other kinds of arthritis, is an inflammation of joints. It attacks the back, particularly the lower back. Aching and stiffness are the primary symptoms, although, like rheumatoid arthritis, it may also produce fever and swelling. Occasionally it appears in the joints of the fingers and toes. We strongly suspect a genetic component in this illness.

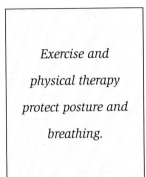

Exercise and physical therapy protect posture and breathing.

Untreated ankylosing spondylitis, through the ravages of inflammation, eventually destroys the bones it attacks. In seeking to heal the inflammation, the body adds fibrous connective tissue and new bone to the affected areas, eventually fusing the bones together and freezing the patient into a permanent, rigid, and often stooping position. The illness is particularly dangerous if the ribs and spine become fused, limiting the patient's ability to breathe.

Physical therapy is very important in treating ankylosing spondylitis. The pain and stiffness make it difficult for patients to carry on their daily activities; it's much easier, I fully understand, to avoid discomfort by moving. But exercise and physical therapy are the best ways to protect your posture and breathing. Daily or more frequent exercise for these purposes is necessary.

The natural medicines that we've already discussed for arthritis will be useful to you. Keep in mind, however, that they don't work right away as pharmaceuticals do. Instead, expect to see changes over time, perhaps three to six weeks. But in the long term you'll have much more benefit from natural remedies than from over-the-counter pain relievers.

FIBROMYALGIA

Q: I was diagnosed as having fibromyalgia. It affects the right side of my face, my eyes, my ear, and my teeth. It's so painful that I can't use my partial plate. I'm wondering what I can do to improve it.

A: Fibromyalgia is a syndrome of muscle pain that has no apparent cause. It is often accompanied by pain in the temporomandibular joint and surrounding tissues, which I suspect is the focus of your problem. A symptom specific to fibromyalgia is "tender points" or "trigger points," small areas where the muscles are very sensitive to touch. While the cause of fibromyalgia is unknown, it is strongly associated with poor sleep, anxiety and/or depression, irritable bowel syndrome, and fatigue. Does any of this pertain to you?

Q: I do have insomnia, and I've felt depressed ever since this problem started. But my digestion seems okay.

> *Sleep difficulties and depression are often intertwined.*

A: Good. Some herbs and natural medicines may well help you overcome your problem. Topical medications that are rubbed on the skin should not be used on the face, and particularly not around the eyes. Instead, I suggest you try some physical therapy with facial exercises and massage; acupuncture may also help.

To promote healing, you should be dealing with your sleep problems. These often are intertwined with depression; it's a vicious circle when you can't get enough sleep, and you feel depressed, and because you're depressed, your sleep isn't refreshing. Address your sleep problems by establishing a relaxing bedtime routine that includes chamomile tea, which is mildly sedative, or extracts or capsules of valerian root, California poppy, or kava kava. Don't take the same herb every time; they are more effective if you vary them.

Deal with your depression by taking St. John's-wort, an herb that has effects similar to those of pharmaceutical antidepressants. Finally, and I know this might seem impossible for you, start an exercise program. Even if you must begin very slowly, exercise to improve your circulation, your outlook, and your overall health.

TEMPOROMANDIBULAR JOINT (TMJ) SYNDROME

Q: I sometimes have a lot of pain in one side of my face, and when I open my mouth there's a thumping sound in the jaw joint. The pain shoots up to my temple, and sometimes down to my collarbone. I'm 43 and in good health otherwise.

A: Are the pain and the noise continuous?

Q: No, it comes and goes, but I don't know why. I have noticed that it occurs mostly during the work week.

A: I suggest that you see your dentist. Your symptoms could be caused by several problems, but I suspect an abscessed tooth or a temporomandibular joint disorder. Both can become gradually troublesome, and both can cause the pain you describe.

Q: If it's TMJ, I'll have to have surgery, right?

A: Not necessarily. Some years ago, surgery was used frequently in cases of TMJ, and often without good results. More conservative and effective therapies ought to be tried before surgery.

The temporomandibular joint, like any other moveable joint in the body, can be damaged by arthritis, overuse, and injury. Most TMJ problems, however, are related to stress. Many folks clench their jaw or grind their teeth as a response to stress, and perhaps grind their teeth at night.

Q: I'm probably one of those people. I'm changing jobs and doing some other things to try to get the stress down in my life.

A: That's great! Too many people lack the courage to take action to alleviate the stress they feel, so they suffer much more than is necessary.

You must get a diagnosis from your dentist or doctor before you start any treatment. If you do have TMJ, use valerian and chamomile for their calming effects, and feverfew as an anti-inflammatory. White willow bark works against pain like aspirin does.

Some patients with TMJ report relief from moist heat applied to the painful area, but others prefer cold packs. Give your jaws a rest by eating foods that require little chewing for a few weeks, and if you can, sleep on your back to rest your shoulder, neck, and facial muscles. The natural therapies of massage, acupuncture, and biofeedback have helped many people with TMJ problems.

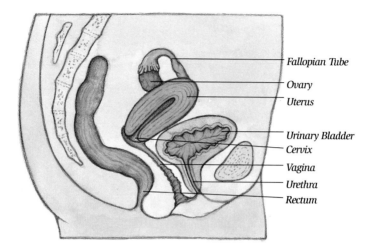

Fallopian Tube

Ovary

Uterus

Urinary Bladder

Cervix

Vagina

Urethra

Rectum

Female Reproductive System

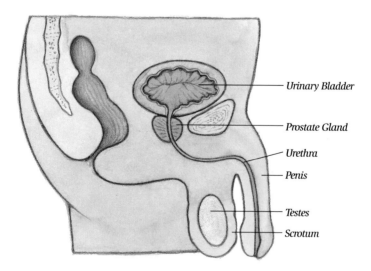

Urinary Bladder

Prostate Gland

Urethra

Penis

Testes

Scrotum

Male Reproductive System

THE REPRODUCTIVE SYSTEM

Good reproductive health is the

foundation of life itself.

The basics of the reproductive system are determined at conception, but nature doesn't finish the job until we approach adulthood. During the preteen or early teen years, the hypothalamus, a gland in the center of the brain, releases a hormone—a chemical messenger—called gonadotropin-releasing hormone (GnRH). Gonads are the reproductive organs—for men the testes, and for women, the ovaries—and "tropin" refers to growth. Thus, the GnRH carries the message, "It's time for the reproductive organs to grow up."

Once released, the hormone travels only a few centimeters to the pituitary gland, which responds by releasing two other hormones that stimulate the gonads. In the male, the gonads respond by producing testosterone and sperm; in the female, the gonads produce estrogen and prompt ovulation. Secondary sexual characteristics also develop. The male develops chest hair, and the female breasts, and the voices of both deepen, although the male's voice gets much lower.

Once sexual maturity is complete, the sexes differ in the consistency of their hormone levels. Men experience a generally even testosterone level throughout their adult lives, and sperm production is relatively constant. While some people debate the existence of a "male menopause," there seems to be no scientific evidence to support its existence.

For women, puberty initiates cycles of fluctuating hormone levels. About every twenty-eight days, the level of estrogen rises and ovulation occurs; then the estrogen level gradually drops and the woman menstruates, but now the level of progesterone is rising. As progesterone peaks and drops again, estrogen begins to rise, leading toward ovulation again. Healthy adult women experience this cycle until menopause.

Even more complex is the hormonal intensity of pregnancy, when all previous patterns change, and change again after birth, and again during lactation. Only when the baby is weaned do the mother's hormones gradually return to the monthly cycle we consider "normal."

Sometime near the age of 50, a woman's estrogen and progesterone levels are reduced, perhaps because the ovaries no longer respond to the chemical messengers. Menstrual cycles typically become shorter and more irregular, and they may occur without ovulation. Eventually, menstruation ceases. This time of decreasing fertility and hormonal adjustment is properly termed the "climacteric," but most people call it "going through menopause." Menopause is reached when menstrual periods have ceased for at least six months. Along with other aspects of women's physiology, these hormonal cycles make the female reproductive system considerably more complex than the male.

STARTING MENSTRUATION EARLY

Q: My sister's little girl is 11, but she has already developed breasts. My sister says she's had her first period. Do you think this is normal, or should she take her daughter to a doctor?

A: First, it's not necessarily a sign of something wrong that the child has started her menstrual cycles. Menstruation can begin anywhere from age 9 to age 16 or 17, so 12 is about average.

> *The average age of first menstruation is twelve.*

It's a good idea for a young girl to have a gynecological exam around the time that she starts her cycles, just to make sure everything is in order. Young girls usually like their mothers to come along, and the mother probably needs to explain the exam to her daughter. Mothers can help by reassuring their daughters that having periods is normal and that this trip to the doctor doesn't mean something is wrong. Is your sister's little girl feeling okay about her situation? Is she having cramps or any other problems?

Q: Her mom said she had a few cramps, but it didn't sound like the daughter really had any problems. I gather it's only happened once, so far.
A: She's probably doing well, then. Your sister may want to schedule an exam for her, to see that everything is normal. It could be done when the girl has her school physical—just add a gynecological exam. I think it's a good idea.

PREMENSTRUAL SYNDROME

Q: I own a small business, and one of my young employees misses a day of work almost every month. A couple of other days she doesn't get much work done. She says she has PMS so bad, she can't get out of bed. What do you think about that? Do you think she's telling the truth? I've had cramps, too, but I never missed work over it.
A: I can't tell if your employee is truthful, of course, but some women do have serious premenstrual symptoms. Debilitating symptoms are rare, but we occasionally see it. How does she describe her problem?

Q: She says she has cramps way up into her back, her legs hurt, and she throws up. At work, she gets depressed and flies off the handle for no reason, and she does swell up quite a bit. She says her breasts hurt, too.
A: All those symptoms are entirely possible. Increased prostaglandin made by the menstrual lining of the uterus is the culprit in most cases of severe PMS. Painful uterine cramps, sometimes spreading into the legs and back, are associated with this hormone, and sometimes we also see intestinal cramping also. That leads to nausea, vomiting, and diarrhea. Stress makes PMS worse.

Your employee first needs a solid diagnosis, because these symptoms could also indicate other problems. Assuming that she does, however, suffer from PMS and nothing else, she can help herself quite a bit without resorting to medications. First, her diet ought to be high in grains, fiber, and fresh fruit and low in fat, especially prior to her period. Fat is hard to digest and contributes to gastrointestinal discomfort; keeping the intestines healthy with good food makes them less likely to cramp. She can supplement with vitamin B against the bloating and mood swings, and try Vitamin E against breast soreness.

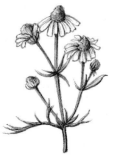

chamomile

Secondly, aerobic exercise, such as walking or swimming, relieves both stress and cramps by releasing endorphins, nature's pain killers—they make you feel good! Stretching exercises and yoga help, too, and she should try meditation and other relaxation techniques. I also can suggest a heating pad on the abdomen, or a hot bath.

For centuries the Chinese have used an herb called dong quai, and this is available in various preparations at natural-food stores. Dong quai balances the hormones and relieves PMS symptoms, sometimes very quickly. Chamomile tea is very relaxing and soothing, too; some recommend soaking a cloth in the tea and applying it to the cramp area. For irritability, a tea made of valerian, cramp bark, and ginger could bring relief.

Q: So you think I shouldn't fire her for being lazy?
A: No, I think her complaints are real. Give her some information and make sure she sees a doctor. If she's a good worker otherwise, she'll appreciate your concern.

CANDIDA

Q: I suffer from recurrent sinus infections, and when I take antibiotics, I get vaginal yeast infections. I've been using over-the-counter medications to get rid of them, but it seems that they come back more and more quickly.
A: Has your doctor diagnosed the yeast infections?

Q: Yes, the first couple of times I had them. They always come on when I take the antibiotics, and I know how they feel and how they're diagnosed. Is there anything I can do to prevent them from recurring?
A: Absolutely. First, the cause of the problem is an imbalance in the natural flora in the vagina, and probably throughout your body. The antibiotics get rid of the bad organisms that cause the infection, but they also kill the good organisms that are needed by your body. Then space becomes

available for other flora to increase, and the yeast organism is one of those that will expand rapidly—it starts having larger families. The antiyeast medications kill some of the yeast, but if you haven't replaced the good organisms, it will return. Then the whole process begins anew.

To remedy the root cause of this yeast problem, take acidophilus. This will balance the flora throughout the body and protect against the overgrowth of yeast. When you must take antibiotics, don't discontinue the acidophilus. Instead, take it two hours before the antibiotic, or two hours after, and keep taking it for several weeks after you finish the antibiotics.

Finally, yeast is encouraged by a diet that is high in refined flours, sugars, and processed foods. Replace these with high-fiber, fresh foods and whole-grain products, and add active-culture yogurt. Then your body will not be such a wonderful environment for candida, and its growth will be limited.

While over-the-counter antiyeast medications are fine to use, they're really a Band-Aid on a bleeding wound. As soon as you take the Band-Aid off, the wound continues bleeding; that is, when you stop using the cream, the yeast returns. But when you take the acidophilus and eat a healthier diet, the problem may heal.

HEALTHY BABIES

Preventing Herpes in Newborns

Q: Is it dangerous to have a baby if you have herpes? Will the baby get it? What natural remedies are helpful for genital herpes?

A: To combat genital herpes, build up your immune system. Herpes is an opportunistic infection, so you are more likely to have an outbreak when the body is weak or debilitated. Keep yourself as healthy as possible by adjusting your diet, exercising, and strengthening your immune system with herbs like echinacea. Put yourself on acidophilus if you haven't already. You could use echinacea during the week before your period and for a few days after.

The supplement L-lysine inhibits the growth of the herpes virus. Also, avoid eating almonds, cashews, and other nuts; barley, meats, dairy products, oats, and grains. Take vitamins A, B complex, and C plus bioflavinoids, as well as the mineral zinc. Reduce stress and otherwise protect your immune system, and when herpes outbreaks do occur, apply tea-tree oil full, strength or diluted with a bland oil, to the sores.

Genital herpes is a sexually transmitted disease that is related to the viruses that cause chickenpox and cold sores. Like those viruses, once genital herpes infects the body, it remains for life. When the immune system is low, the virus can erupt again, first causing itching, soreness, and perhaps flu-like symptoms, and then painful lesions in the genital area. The following circular sores take up to ten days to heal. The first outbreak, which comes seven to ten days after exposure, is for most people the most painful and intense. Complications occur infrequently but can include liver inflammation, nerve damage, and meningitis. The antiviral medications Zovirax and Acyclovir reduce the severity of outbreaks but don't prevent them entirely.

With regard to having a baby, we once believed that if the mother had genital herpes, the baby must be delivered by Cesarean section to avoid the possibility of infection as it passes through the birth canal. This precaution was taken for good reason: In infants, this herpes virus can cause blindness, brain damage, and death. Now, however, by taking oral medications, most women with herpes can have regular vaginal deliveries, and their babies are safe.

If the mother has no active lesions, a vaginal birth is just as possible for her as for an uninfected person. Because the lesions can be hidden internally, a thorough vaginal exam should be made by a competent professional immediately before the patient gives birth. Cesarean section remains the only recourse if lesions are present. You should talk to your obstetrician, of course, but genital herpes does not mean you shouldn't have a baby.

Spina Bifida

Q: There's spina bifida in my family, so I'm concerned about having children.

A: In the first trimester of pregnancy, probably the fifth or sixth week, the delicate spinal cord of the fetus typically becomes encased by the bones of the spine. If the spine does not close, spina bifida results; the spinal cord protrudes through the opening, sometimes even extending outside the body. Spinal cord damage and consequent disability are inevitable, but degrees of damage vary greatly depending on the extent of the injury. The lower on the spine the damage occurs, the less disability. Sometimes we see decreased mental capacity with spina bifida.

Spina bifida can be diagnosed during pregnancy, most accurately by amniocentesis. Some doctors use blood tests and ultrasounds later in pregnancy. No evidence exists that spina bifida is genetic.

Q: That's pretty scary.
A: I agree, but we have good news about preventing spina bifida. Seventy percent of the incidences of spina bifida can be prevented by ensuring that pregnant women receive adequate folic acid. And because spina bifida occurs so early in pregnancy—perhaps before the woman even knows she is pregnant—anyone anticipating pregnancy should start taking a good multivitamin, available over the counter, that contains adequate folic acid. Young women over age 15 should have 180 micrograms daily, but pregnant women should receive 400 micrograms, and nursing mothers need 280 micrograms.

Folate deficiency is common among people who consume few fresh vegetables. Folic acid is deteriorated by light and heat, and many prescription medications disrupt its utilization by the body. Yet it is essential to proper cell division and the development of the nervous system. Folate deficiency is also implicated in depression, atherosclerosis, osteoporosis, and other illnesses.

> *Seventy percent of spina bifida cases can be prevented.*

Foods high in folic acid include brewer's yeast; green, leafy vegetables such as spinach and kale; garbanzos and most beans; and walnuts, asparagus, and other familiar vegetables. Folic acid or folate supplements providing up to 400 micrograms daily are available; folinic acid is the most active form. Folate supplements should include vitamin B_{12} (400 to 1,000 mcg daily).

Amenorrhea

Q: I'm in my twenties, and my husband and I would like to have a child. But I'm also a dancer and a runner, and I stopped having menstrual cycles a couple of years ago, probably because I'm so thin, my doctor says.

I've been trying to gain weight, in hopes that the cycles will start again, but so far they haven't. Is there anything else I can do?

A: Amenorrhea—the absence of menstrual cycles—can be caused by the ratio of body fat to overall weight falling too low. So the problem isn't how much you weigh, but how much of the food you take into your body can be stored in reserve versus how much is used right away or turned into muscle. Nature prevents pregnancy when the mother doesn't have enough nutrients to sustain another life. Are you still running and dancing?

Q: Yes. I've been trying to add more calories to my diet.
A: Has your doctor recommended that you cut back on the exercise?

Q: Well, yes. But it's very hard to give that up.
A: You like those endorphins! But you may have to choose between giving up some of your running and dancing for a while and having a child. As long as you continue rigorous exercise, your body will find it difficult to set aside calories as fat.

Fat is your body's savings account: you can put calories into fat only if you have some left over after all your metabolic bills are paid. And if you continue exercising, the bills are going to stay high. All that energy has to come from someplace, and it's coming from the food you eat. If you convert all of your food into energy, none remains to become fat. I don't mean you should stop exercising entirely—you shouldn't. But you may have to cut back if you want to regain your fertility.

Q: Are there any herbal products that stimulate the menstrual cycles?
A: Some herbal therapies that are used to normalize the hormones, such as dong quai. Herbs alone, however, probably can't restart your menses unless you also increase your amount of body fat.

BREAST HEALTH

Breast Cyst
Q: I have a cyst in my breast, and my doctor wants to do a biopsy. If it's just a cyst, do I really need a biopsy? Can a cyst in the breast become cancerous, or cause other kinds of problems?

A: I feel very strongly that every woman over 40 should have an annual mammogram, regardless of the recommendations of national commissions or other broad pronouncements. Anyone who finds a thickening or lump in the breast should have one immediately. If the mammogram shows a cyst, certainly a biopsy is warranted. Most breast cysts are of minor concern, but if the biopsy shows hyperplasia—an unusual increase in the number of cells in that tissue—the cyst will have a higher likelihood of becoming cancer than an ordinary cyst. It should be watched very closely. Dysplasia—cells that are abnormal in size, shape, and organization—is also detected by biopsy. Certainly if dysplasia is occurring, you need to know about it.

Another cause for concern is microcalcifications. In the mammogram, they look like grains of pepper in the breast. A biopsy should be done as there is a higher likelihood of cancer in that area, too.

Q: Is dysplasia associated with cancer?
A: Yes, especially in cervical cancers, which are usually reported as dysplasia. For women with breast discomfort and fibrocystic disease, we've found that good breast health is promoted by eliminating coffee, tea, cola, and chocolate from the diet for at least a month. Also, focus your diet on vegetables, eliminate fats, and eat lots of high-fiber foods such as whole-wheat and bran products. You're also likely to benefit from eating lots of dark-green, leafy vegetables and bright yellow vegetables such as carrots and sweet potatoes.

Breast Cancer

Q: When my wife had her breast removed, a lump was discovered on her left lung, and her doctor recommended radiation therapy. Can she have some other treatment, like chemotherapy pills, so she doesn't have to go through radiation?
A: Yes, she can try other treatments. Before you make the decision to go another direction, however, please learn more about today's radiation treatments. Years ago, radiation treatments for cancer involved a large area of the body, which meant that folks got a high dose and suffered very unpleasant side effects. Now, using focused beam radiation, doctors can identify the best way to attack the cancer, mark the skin very pre-

cisely, and irradiate a much smaller area. The patient has a much easier time of it than previously.

Oral chemotherapy may not be so effective for your wife as radiation. Discuss various treatment options with an oncologist, who will help you consider all the factors as you make the decision: the type of cancer, the type of cells, and whether they are estrogen-receptor positive or progesterone-receptor positive. The best decision for your wife is one that is informed and thoughtful and made with the help of your doctor.

Q: Do you know of any herbs that might help her?
A: If your wife is overweight, she should lose the excess. The body's fat tends to store extra hormones, and that could influence tumor development. And of course she should eat only minimal amounts of fat and eliminate it completely if she can. Fiber in her diet is very important; she should eat apples, dried beans prepared without fat, oatmeal, and bran products. The dark green and bright yellow vegetables, such as leaf lettuce and winter squash, are good for her. Also, garlic, tofu, and kelp.

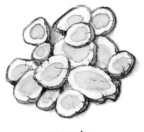
astragalus

The herbs astragalus and burdock may help your wife. Astragalus stimulates immunity and is believed to help heal cancer; it acts as an adaptogen to normalize tissue and is particularly beneficial when taken along with ginseng. Burdock root purifies the blood; simmer a piece of the root in water and drink as a tea or use in sauces. It is a great body cleanser. Supplement with vitamins A (beta carotene), C plus bioflavinoids, and E.

MENOPAUSE

As women age, estrogen levels decline. First comes a transitional period called perimenopause; menopause itself commences when no menstruation has occurred for six months. As hormonal levels decline, many women experience hot flashes, night sweats, mood changes, and flushing in varying degrees of severity. Disturbed sleep produces additional fatigue and irritability. Temporary memory loss, dizziness, and heart palpitations are commonly reported. Nonetheless, a few women pass through menopause with few symptoms.

Menopause occurs suddenly for women whose ovaries are removed or cease to function. Radiation, chemotherapy, and surgery are the most likely causes of abrupt menopause, although unexplained early menopause is associated with smoking. These women do not have the luxury of the gradual cessation of fertility; instead, they immediately feel the full force of drastically lowered hormonal levels. All women experiencing menopause, regardless of when it occurs, are at increased risk for osteoporosis and heart disease.

Sudden Menopause

Q: I've had my ovaries removed because of cancer, and I'm having hot flashes and all those symptoms. I can't have estrogen because of the kind of tumor I had, and I'm wondering if there are any natural remedies that will help me.
A: Black cohosh could help you with the menopausal hot flashes and night sweats. In Europe, it is often successfully prescribed for precisely the symptoms you describe. The Chinese herb dong quai is used in traditional remedies for menstrual and menopausal difficulties. It normalizes estrogen levels. Do you sleep well?

Q: Well, no. I wake up at night and throw the covers off because I'm too hot. Then I start worrying about my cancer recurring.
A: St. John's-wort or valerian could help you sleep and get a handle on your anxiety. Both are quite effective in promoting relaxation and a good night's sleep. Gotu kola may also help in this regard.

Adjust your diet to include mostly fruits and vegetables and whole-grain products. Don't eat dairy products, sugar, or anything containing caffeine. Because hot foods like soup or spicy foods can bring on hot flashes, avoid them. Instead, eat plenty of soybeans, tofu, miso, flaxseed, pomegranates, and dates. Kombucha tea also eases menopausal symptoms.

Osteoporosis and Menopause

Q: I'm approaching menopause and getting worried about my bones softening due to osteoporosis. Are the antacids that I see advertised a good calcium supplement?

A: No, you need much more calcium than antacids provide, and you are right to be concerned about the health of your bones. Lower estrogen levels in your body will allow bone loss, which begins for most women in the mid thirties, to accelerate. Osteoporosis is a serious threat; not only is it painful, but the broken bones of someone with osteoporosis heal poorly.

I suggest vitamins E, D, and K to slow the aging process. Supplements of calcium of up to 1,500 milligrams per day are needed, along with 1,000 milligrams of magnesium to make sure the body takes up the calcium properly. Select calcium citrate, calcium gluconate, or calcium lactate. The usual form, calcium carbonate, is difficult to for the body to use. The supplement L-lysine aids calcium absorption.

More important, however, is the role of weight-bearing exercise in keeping the bones strong. Walking, weight-lifting, and similar exercises help the body strengthen the vertebrae, the long bones, and the pelvis. Without exercise, your plan for protecting the bones is simply incomplete.

Memory Loss During Menopause

Q: I'm going through menopause, and I'm getting along with it pretty well, but I really can't stand forgetting things all the time. I know it's normal and temporary, but I just hate it.

A: Are you taking hormone replacement therapy?

Q: No. My mother had a very easy menopause, so I thought I'd try it without the hormones. Except for this one problem I'm doing okay.

A: Good! You could try some Siberian ginseng. Studies have shown that it improves both physical and mental performance under stress, so it might be helpful for the fatigue and fuzzy-mindedness that sometimes go along with menopause. Ginkgo biloba and blue cohosh may also help.

Estrogen Deficiency

Q: I'm not quite forty yet, but about a year ago I started having several seemingly unrelated problems, and now it looks like they were all related to a lower-than-usual level of estrogen.

A: What kinds of symptoms were you having?

Q: Well, moodiness, especially around my periods, less interest in sex, and vaginal dryness. I had recurrent bladder infections and then gardnerella, a vaginal infection. I was using a cervical cap for birth control, and I noticed that my cervix seemed to be protruding more than usual—this really scared me, because I thought it might be cervical cancer. When I went for my gynecological exam, the doctor said all this was related to estrogen deficiency. I was surprised that estrogen deficiency could do so much.

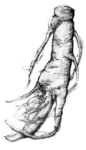

ginseng

A: Estrogen deficiency can cause your infection problems because it affects the pH—the level of acidity or alkalinity—in your system. If the body's pH changes, it allows bacteria that are usually controlled to grow. The gardnerella, which is a nonspecific vaginal infection, could have proliferated because of this change.

The cervical protrusion is caused by a relaxing of the muscle tone of your uterus and vagina. Estrogen plays a major role in keeping those tissues in good condition, which is probably why you're getting the vaginal dryness now. Did you have any blood work done to give you a definite diagnosis?

Q: No. The doctor did what he called a "cell maturity index," which showed that yes, my estrogen level has dropped.
A: So what are your questions?

Q: I tried a birth control pill to raise the estrogen level. At first I felt quite a bit better, but now, after eight months, it's not so effective, and I'm getting headaches. I was wondering if herbs that contain phytoestrogens would be effective. Also, would I still need to take progesterone to balance them, the way they say I should with the chemical estrogen replacements. And why do women with their uterus still in place have to balance with progesterone?
A: The progesterone protects you against cancer of the breast, ovaries, and uterus. It is important to continue taking it. To help the symptoms of low estrogen, try extracts of wild yam and damiana, and perhaps dong quai also.

The big question, of course, is why your ovaries are not producing enough estrogen. You should schedule a visit with your doctor to discuss that question.

Chlorine and Menopause

Q: I've heard that chlorine can cause problems for menopausal women. My mother is going through menopause, and she swims a lot. Is this a good idea?

A: Chlorine mimics the sex hormone estrogen, which has been linked to various forms of breast cancer. High levels of chlorine are also linked to colon and bladder cancer. Consequently, we want to limit exposure to chlorine, especially if other risk factors are present. This is true for men as well as women. Although we usually see a very low incidence of breast cancer in men—less than one percent—I had two male patients in 1995 with breast cancer.

For most people, the primary source of chlorine exposure is household water from the public supply. During a twenty-minute shower, for instance, the body absorbs the amount of chlorine in a gallon of water. Swimming in a chlorinated pool or soaking in a chlorinated hot tub certainly increases that basic exposure.

Protect yourself from chlorine by using water filters.

In addition to mimicking estrogen, chlorine triggers bronchospasm. I myself am particularly aware of that when I use the hot tub at a public pool because I come out wheezing. You can protect yourself from chlorine in household water by using water-filtering devices; some are made to fit over your shower head at home.

Chlorine in the water is one of the areas targeted in an ongoing Columbia University study of the high incidence of breast cancer on Long Island. Researchers believe that the soil or the water may hold clues to this problem, so they are studying pesticides and herbicides too.

Hormone Replacement Therapy

Q: Years ago, there was a big scare about estrogen causing breast cancer. My mother refused to take hormones because of it. Now I hear that estrogen is safe, so I'm considering taking it. Is this okay?

A: Earlier forms of hormone replacement therapy (HRT) did not include progesterone. Some studies associated the therapy with increased ovarian and breast cancer. The present forms of HRT that combine estrogen and progesterone, however, are quite safe.

Hormone replacement therapy, often prescribed for menopausal women, supplements the body's declining hormones with various forms of estrogen and progesterone. Although many women experience unpleasant side effects, such as indigestion, from today's HRT, it also has distinct benefits. Studies show that HRT helps protect the cardiovascular system and can prevent heart disease and osteoporosis. If you're interested in the therapy, discuss the details with your doctor. It may be a good choice for you.

INCONTINENCE

Q: Are there any herbs to help with incontinence?
A: In men, we need to make sure there isn't an infection or a prostate problem. And in women, we need to rule out both infection and uterine and bladder problems. So the first thing to do is to see a urologist or gynecologist. Get a good checkup.

As for treatment, if infection is a factor in your incontinence try cranberry supplements to prevent and treat it. Cranberries don't change the acidity of the urine. Instead, they contain an anti-adherence factor; so bacteria can't stick to the bladder wall. They can't create infection.

For women, Kegel exercises are excellent for improving control of the bladder. Named for the person who invented them, Kegel exercises strengthen the wide muscle, the pubococcygeus (PC), that stretches from the pubic bone to the tail bone. It supports all the organs located in the pelvis, including the uterus, the bladder, and the lower colon. Like other muscles, it can become weak without exercise. Then you face the likelihood of prolapsed uterus, urinary incontinence, and less pleasurable sex.

Exercising the PC muscle increases pelvic circulation, strengthens the muscle, and increases the ability to control the bladder. The exercises are easy: the PC muscle is the one used to delay urination and to tighten the anus. Concentrate on tightening and releasing the muscle as you sit, stand, or drive, and count the repetitions. Work up slowly to about 200 per day to effectively control urinary incontinence.

MEN'S REPRODUCTIVE HEALTH

Prostate Health

The prostate gland is located at the base of the male's urinary bladder and is wrapped around the urethra. This gland produces the fluid in which the sperm are suspended at the time of ejaculation.

Typically, the prostate gland is about the size of a walnut, but with increasing age nearly all men experience prostate enlargement or benign prostatic hypertrophy (BPH). According to the American College of Urology, BPH affects 27 million American men. Half of 50-year-old men and 80 percent of 80-year-old men have it.

The symptoms of BPH are quite familiar to older men. Because the enlarged prostate squeezes the urethra, urination becomes disrupted. Getting up at night, frequent urination, uneven urine flow, and urgency are the usual symptoms of BPH.

Unfortunately, along with blood in the urine, painful urination, and continuing lower back or pelvic pain, these are also symptoms of prostate cancer. Distinguishing a benign inflammation of the prostate from prostate cancer requires an examination by a urologist. Even one of these symptoms warrants a prompt visit. To further complicate matters, prostate cancer can show no symptoms at all until it is advanced; this makes annual exams for men over 50 very important.

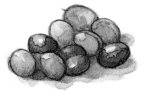

saw palmetto

Doctors most frequently recommend surgery to treat BPH; ten percent of men will have at least one prostate surgery. There are alternatives to surgery, however: preparations of saw palmetto, pygeum, and zinc are very helpful in treating BPH. Men lose zinc as they age, and the prostate needs it. If deprived of zinc, the prostate is susceptible to swelling and inflammation. In many cases, zinc supplements reduce prostate swelling significantly.

Prostate-Specific Antigen Test (PSA)

Q: A friend's doctor says he needs a PSA test. What is it?

A: When the prostate gland is enlarged, it releases a chemical called prostate-specific antigen (PSA). Usually we see the PSA level at zero to four. If the PSA is between four and ten, the health of the prostate needs further investigation. Hence the PSA test.

While the incidence of cancer seems to increase with the PSA level, much more information is needed to diagnose cancer. I've seen men with PSAs of five who have prostate cancer, and some with PSAs of fifteen with enlarged prostates but no cancer. Infection can elevate the PSA, too. The PSA is just one diagnostic tool among several that are used when the prostate is enlarged. Your friend shouldn't worry until more tests are required.

Preventing Prostate Problems

Q: I really don't want to develop prostate problems. Is there anything you can recommend?

A: Absolutely. If you care for your prostate well, your prostate will take care of you. You can prevent prostate disease instead of trying to reverse it later. I suggest to my patients that they take saw palmetto with pygeum, and supplement with zinc. You might also consider taking the amino acids glycine, alanine, and glutamic acid. Saw palmetto, however, is a phenomenal preventive, and combined with the pygeum and the zinc, it's excellent.

IMPOTENCE

Q: I'm 51, and I seem to be developing a problem with impotence. Two or three times in the last six months I've had this trouble.

A: That's not unusual, you know. Studies have shown that slightly over half the men in your age group have impotence from time to time. Are you in good health otherwise? Do you smoke or drink?

Q: I quit smoking years ago, and I do drink a glass of beer now and then. My wife and I like a drink on our special evenings. I have gastroesophageal reflux disorder—GERD—and I take an over-the-counter medication for that, two every morning.

A: What medication do you take?

Q: Zantac or Tagamet, usually. Whichever is cheaper; they both help my stomach.

A: Congratulations on quitting smoking. But did you know that alcohol can interfere with your sexual ability?

Q: Really? I thought it was good because it's relaxing and pleasant.
A: That can be true also, but alcohol decreases your testosterone level, and that's the hormone that encourages sexual interest. Avoid alcohol in general, and particularly when your are anticipating sex.

The medications you are taking for your stomach have also been implicated in decreased sexual desire and impotence, so you should consult your doctor about finding an alternative medication. Certainly don't stop taking your medication without your doctor's approval. Other medications that are used to treat high blood pressure, antidepressants, and stimulants have been identified as interfering with sexual function also.

Q: Do you think it could be a psychological problem?
A: You could answer that better than I, but here's an easy test. If you have erections at night or early in the morning, you probably don't have a physical problem, and a psychological evaluation could be helpful. If you don't have nighttime erections, a physical problem is more likely.

If this problem persists, your doctor should give you a careful examination for thyroid, cardiovascular, and endocrine problems such as diabetes. Disorders in these areas are proven to produce impotence.

For occasional problems such as you describe, however, avoid the alcohol and check with your doctor for a different stomach medication. In addition, an excellent diet that is low in fats will help your overall health. Zinc supplements, vitamin E, and saw palmetto may also improve the health of your reproductive system.

The herb damiana improves circulation in the genital area, and the steroids contained in wild yam may invigorate your performance. A tea of dong quai also normalizes the hormones and may help you. You'll also find numerous commercial preparations in the health store that claim to stimulate sexual performance, and some have benefited from them.

Q: I'm 76 years old, not on any medication, and had a prostate exam about a year ago with no problems indicated. But I have difficulty maintaining an erection. Are there any herbs that will help?
A: How long since you've seen your doctor for a complete exam?

Q: Well, quite a while, but I've been healthy. So I haven't gone.
A: You need to see your doctor to make sure you're healthy through and through. Are you taking zinc or any other dietary supplements?

Q: No.
A: It might be good for you to start taking zinc, then, because it is essential to the health of the prostate. Then follow up with vitamin E. Herbs that have been traditionally used to increase staying power are wild yam and damiana. You might give them a try.

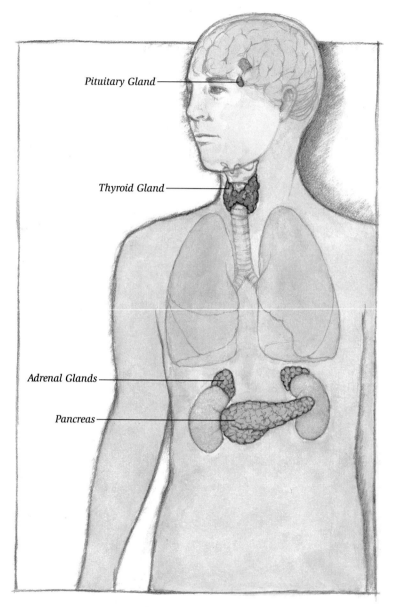

Pituitary Gland

Thyroid Gland

Adrenal Glands

Pancreas

The Endocrine System

THE ENDOCRINE SYSTEM

The glands allow us to adapt to our changing

experiences and environment.

A complex network of glands and tissue, the endocrine system performs innumerable physical tasks by secreting tiny amounts of hormones that stimulate change and adjustment in various parts of the body. Each hormone functions in specific ways to keep the body functioning smoothly and in balance. Every organ and system is influenced by them. The hormones are most notably involved with the maturation and function of the reproductive system, growth, the use of nutrients in the body, and balancing the body's fluids. An efficiently operating endocrine system usually goes unnoticed, but a malfunctioning one can create drastic problems.

The interactions of the parts of the endocrine system are subtle yet powerful; our most essential bodily functions depend upon the signals that originate in the endocrine glands. For instance, during late pregnancy the hypothalamus, located in the base of the brain, induces labor when gestation is complete; linked to the hypothalamus, the pituitary gland stimulates the breasts to produce milk. Later, the child's pituitary produces muscle and bone growth, and, during puberty, initiates the maturation of the sexual organs and production of sperm or eggs. A failure of any of these processes is considered a serious health crisis.

The most common endocrine disorder is diabetes mellitus, which occurs when the body is unable to properly use insulin, or when insulin is not produced within the pancreas. Other disorders created by endocrine disruption are premature puberty or failure to achieve puberty, certain types of infertility, lactation unassociated with pregnancy, thyroid dysfunction including goiter, certain kinds of mental retardation, rapid heart beat, and frequent sweating.

Although scientific research uncovers new information about the endocrine system regularly, it remains poorly understood. The precise function of specific glands and hormones, the range of their impact, and the subtlety of hormonal and glandular interactions remain mysterious.

DIABETES

Diabetes mellitus afflicts about sixteen million Americans, but only half are diagnosed and receiving treatment. An unknown additional number have early, unrecognized glucose intolerance that may lead to diabetes. The disorder occurs when the body's cells cannot correctly use glucose derived from carbohydrates and instead fuel themselves primarily with protein and fats.

Insulin, a hormone, is the key factor in diabetes mellitus. In a healthy person, specialized cells in the pancreas produce adequate, functional insulin that binds with the body's cells and allows them to receive and burn glucose derived from ingested carbohydrates and some protein. When something interferes with this process, diabetes occurs. We don't know exactly what disrupts the glucose-burning process. Some theorize that a virus may trigger the problem, and others believe that the body's immune system somehow attacks the insulin, the cells, or both, making glucose use difficult or impossible.

Type 1 diabetes is typically diagnosed during childhood but certainly before the patient reaches thirty years of age. These diabetics tend to be slender because the beta-2 cells of the pancreas don't make enough insulin to transport sugar into the cells, so the body turns to its fats for energy. About ten percent of diabetics are Type 1.

Type 2 diabetes occurs when the body's cells cannot use insulin effectively, whether or not enough is produced. Type 2 diabetes is far more prevalent than Type 1, and it primarily affects those overweight people in the later part of life. Type II diabetics are usually not insulin-dependent, though they may at some point need insulin to control their blood-sugar levels.

The main symptoms of diabetes are frequent urination, excessive and unexplained thirst, unexplained weight loss, and frequent hunger. Some patients also report fatigue, headaches, irritability, lethargy, blurred vision, itching, or slow healing.

Whichever type of diabetes the individual has, the outcome of untreated diabetes is a dangerous condition that affects every organ and system in the body.

Regulating Blood Sugar

Q: I'm a Type I diabetic, and I take insulin. I wonder what alternative medicine has to offer.
A: Do you have a good relationship with your physician?

Q: Yes. I feel I've gotten good guidance from her—certainly my health has improved. I just wonder if there's more I should be doing.
A: Are you exercising?

Q: I walk several miles daily, and sometimes I go to the gym and work out on the weight machines.
A: That sounds very good. Exercise is essential to your control of your condition. Diabetes is complicated, and right now we can't cure it. If your physician agrees, you can try chromium picolinate to help regulate your blood-sugar level. The chromium makes the insulin more effective. You might also consider vitamin B complex plus biotin and inositol to boost your glucose metabolism.

Your diet should include very few fats. Instead eat a high-fiber diet that includes many vegetables, berries, low-fat dairy products, eggs, fish, and garlic. Soybean products such as tofu provide protein, as do combinations of legumes and nuts, so these are better for you than meat.

Because diabetics have a predisposition to yeast infections, I recommend you take acidophilus. Yeast thrives in warm, dark, environments and is encouraged by the presence of sugars. Diabetics have a greater number of skin infections from yeast; women may get them underneath the breasts and in the groin areas. Diabetic men may get athlete's foot as well as groin infections. Therefore, acidophilus becomes very important to prevent skin problems and digestive ones, too.

When you're trying to get control of your diabetes, you need a comprehensive program that you and your physician develop together. It's crucial, if you're going to try any herbs or supplements along with insulin, that you consult with your physician. It is very dangerous to try to regulate your own insulin or to take any action that may interfere with it.

Glucose Testing

Q: How often do I really need to test my blood sugar? My diabetes isn't that bad; I don't have to take insulin.

A: The Diabetes Control and Complication Trial, a comprehensive ten-year study of 14,000 diabetics, recommends that diabetics check their blood glucose four times a day. If you want to be a purist with very sore fingers, that's what you can do.

A more practical method is to use a two-day cycle of testing. On Day 1, test yourself in the morning, one half hour before breakfast, and test again in the evening, one half hour before dinner. On Day 2, take a test one half hour before lunch, and again at bedtime. This cycle of tests will give you a good cross-section of your glucose levels. From this information, your doctor will be able to determine how to regulate your insulin.

Childhood Diabetes

Q: Have you any suggestions about natural medicine for a three-year-old boy recently diagnosed with diabetes?

A: You and your family must work very closely with his physician to learn about your child's illness and how to take care of him. Childhood diabetes is a challenge for everyone in the family, and if your physician is not counseling you about the problems you and your child are likely to face, you may want to find a psychologist with experience in this area. I also recommend a support group for families of children with diabetes. Many hospitals and community organizations offer such groups. Your child's success in coping with his illness throughout his life depends on early intervention and how well you teach him to take over the management of his illness.

To help your child, first be sure that his diet is healthy. Fats, sugars, and refined flours are out. He also needs to have regular exercise, and his glucose levels must be monitored. In a child so young, I recommend that you discuss your interest in natural medicine with his physician.

Dietary Cautions

Q: I'm a diabetic, and I'd like to take beta carotene to improve my health. Is there any problem with this?

A: It would be better for you to take an emulsion of vitamin A because it's difficult for diabetics to convert beta carotene into the A. Also, some research indicates that the amino acid cysteine and large doses of vitamins B_1, B_3, and C interfere with insulin absorption, and you don't need that. Don't take any of these supplements without getting the approval of your physician.

Preventing Diabetes

Q: There is diabetes in my family. What can I do to avoid getting it myself?

A: There is no guaranteed way of avoiding diabetes, but research indicates that Type 2 diabetes is somehow linked with the same conditions that foster cardiovascular disease. Therefore, you may be able to prevent Type II diabetes by keeping your weight in the normal range, exercising regularly, and eating a diet that promotes heart health. That is, your diet should be low in fats, high in fiber, and contain no refined sugar or white flour.

Your annual checkup should include blood-sugar monitoring. You should also have a yearly eye examination, and your physician should check your feet at each regular examination. Changes in the eyes and sensitivity of the feet can signal early diabetes, which is more easily treated if diagnosed before it causes severe damage.

THE COMPLICATIONS OF DIABETES

The impact of diabetes is felt throughout the body; no system escapes the problems that occur when cells cannot function normally. The complications an individual may face, or the degree of severity, is difficult to predict. Sometimes complications appear suddenly, and sometimes they appear years or even decades after the diabetes is diagnosed. Even patients who faithfully test and regulate their blood sugar can experience problems, but those who neglect the illness are almost certain to have great difficulties. According the Diabetes Control and Complications Trial, the better you control your diabetes, the more likely you are to stay healthy and avoid serious complications.

Dealing with these complications often becomes as great a concern as controlling the diabetes itself, for the complications can become disabling or even life-threatening. As a consequence, it's important for diabetics to stay in close contact with their physician and to report problems even though they seem minor and unrelated to the diabetes.

Neuropathy

Neuropathy, a complication of diabetes, starts very early in the progression of diabetes. It may result when blood sugar reaches too high a level and interferes with nerve conduction. Some of the typical symptoms are tingling and numbness of the feet or fingers, unexplained pain, slowed reflexes, and sexual impotence. In more advanced cases of neuropathy, all sensation is lost in a particular area.

Diabetic neuropathy is the primary cause of nontraumatic limb loss in this country. Eighty percent of amputations that are not caused by vehicle accidents or other traumas are the result of diabetes. Typically these amputations become necessary because the limb has been injured. Due to the fact that the patient could not feel the injury, the wound was neglected, became badly infected, and had to be removed. Sometimes the cardiovascular complications of diabetes interfere with circulation to the limbs, and amputation becomes necessary for that reason.

Gastroparesis

Q: I'm a Type II diabetic. I've developed some unpleasant problems with my digestion—constipation, gas, and so on.
A: Diabetics can develop a condition known as gastroparesis, and it has to do with the nerve damage they can experience. The nerves that control intestinal motility—the movement that forces food to move through the intestine—are damaged, so the movement slows. The antibiotic erythromycin can stimulate the intestine to get moving again, but it has side effects like stomach upset and diarrhea, so I don't particularly recommend it.

Instead, I recommend that you try aloe vera gel, which is exceptional for softening the stools and gently stimulating movement in the intestine. You can also make the intestine's job easier by taking fiber. Psyllium husk is excellent; if you do not now eat a high-fiber diet, begin with about a quarter dose (according to the manufacturer's directions) and gradually increase to a full dose. Finally, acidophilus will help keep your intestine healthy and prevent an overgrowth of candida, or yeast. And be sure to report this digestive problem to your doctor.

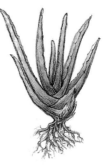

aloe vera

Sore Feet

Q: I'm a diabetic. What herbs can I take for my feet, which burn and tingle and get red and inflamed? Also for blood pressure. One doctor called my problems osteoarthritis.

A: The foot inflammation may be from peripheral neuropathy, a deadening of the nerves in the extremities. Diabetes somehow interferes with the ability of the nerves to communicate pain or discomfort, and the symptoms are as you describe. A person without diabetes will shift position when a foot goes to sleep, but a diabetic with damaged nerves won't feel that sensation. Likewise, a little sore on a diabetic's foot can become a serious problem, even lead to amputation, because the diabetic can't feel the pain that another person would.

There's a simple test for neuropathy in the feet: ask someone to lightly brush your toes with a very fine brush while you close your eyes. If you can feel the brushing, there is no neuropathy present. If you can't, you are at risk for developing foot ulcers and sores. A visit with a podiatrist is important. Also, diabetics ought not to clip their own toenails because if the skin is nicked, it will not heal well. Always wear shoes or slippers for the same reason.

Are there herbs to help your feet? To strengthen your blood vessels and stimulate your cardiovascular system, I recommend hawthorn and garlic. Ginkgo biloba, butchers broom root, and cayenne also stimulate the circulation. Most important, however, is completely protecting your feet by always wearing shoes or slippers.

Retinopathy

Q: Why do you tell your diabetic patients that they must have their eyes checked every year? Does diabetes affect the eyes?

A: Diabetes is the number one cause of nontraumatic blindness in this country. An ophthalmologist is trained and equipped to recognize early signs of retinopathy, the deterioration of the eye's retina, or viewing screen, that can be a complication of diabetes. Early cataracts also go along with diabetes; the clear lens in the front of the eye becomes cloudy. That's why visits to the eye doctor are so important for diabetics.

These changes in the eye are actually a result of weakened blood vessels that serve the retina. The vessels may leak blood into the retina, or they may die and leave an area unnourished and unable to function. Sometimes a tiny vessel bursts, and the fluid inside the eye, the vitreous humor, is stained until the body reabsorbs the blood.

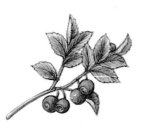

bilberry

For my diabetic patients, I recommend supporting the health of the eyes with bilberry, which can be taken as an extract. The herb eyebright is also beneficial as a tea. Herbs that help strengthen the blood vessels include hawthorn, ginkgo biloba, and garlic.

Cardiovascular Disease

Q: My mother says she's had a "silent heart attack." She didn't even know about it, had no symptoms at all, but her doctor said it happened. Is that possible? She's in her mid-sixties, and she's a diabetic, but she doesn't seem to have too many problems from the diabetes.

A: Your mom may well have had a heart attack just as she described. Diabetics can have "silent heart attacks" because the nerves that signal heart disease are impaired by the diabetes. These people don't have the various types of pain that most heart-attack victims describe, but they have heart attacks just the same.

Circulatory problems are very typical of diabetics. More than other patients, diabetics tend to develop hardening of the arteries—fat deposits in the blood vessels—and high blood pressure. Hawthorn is an excellent herb for strengthening the circulation. Ginkgo is a vasodilator, so it helps the circulation in tiny blood vessels. Garlic is also very good for circulation; it allows the blood to flow smoothly. Vitamin B_1, or thiamine, or a good B complex with vitamin B_6 are all very good, but take no more than the recommended dosage. Please encourage your mother to work close-ly with her physician to limit the complications of her diabetes.

Nephropathy

One of the most important tests for diabetics is the urine test for microalbuminurea, an early predictor of diabetic kidney disease. Albumin is a component of protein, and it appears in the urine when kidney disease is present. Kidney disease can accelerate very quickly and must be brought under control. Even transplanted kidneys do not stay healthy if the diabetic cannot or does not con-trol the diabetes. Controlling blood pressure and blood sugar minimize the damage of diabetes to the kidneys.

Kidney disease is a common problem for diabetics.

Q: What is the latest treatment for Syndrome X?
A: Syndrome X was described ten or fifteen years ago as a pattern that includes diabetes, high blood pressure, and hyperlipidemia, or high triglyceride levels. The syndrome is connected in some way with insulin resistance, a confusing situation in which the body produces insulin, but the cells can't or won't take it up.

Weight management is the key to resolving Syndrome X, although we don't know exactly how diabetes and obesity are linked. We do know that a healthy diet eases the symptoms of Syndrome X. Some new oral medications regulate glucose levels through the liver, and others work through carbohydrate metabolism. They can be taken along with insulin to try to resolve Syndrome X.

THYROID DISEASE

The thyroid gland, which sits above the larynx, or voice box, in the throat, secretes thyroid hormone. It regulates how quickly the body burns calories. The thyroid requires regular intake of iodine to function correctly. Without iodine, the thyroid enlarges to a goiter and malfunctions.

A thyroid gland that is overactive produces too much hormone, creating a hypERthyroid condition with symptoms such as nervousness, anxiety, weight loss, excessive sweating, and intolerance to heat. Every body process speeds up, resulting in malabsorption and other complications. A thyroid gland that is underactive produces too little thyroid, and that's called hypOthyroidism. Symptoms are constipation, hair loss, fatigue, lethargy, and intolerance to cold. Hypothyroidism is more common than hyperthyroidism and is usually treated with synthetic thyroid hormone.

The cause of many thyroid malfunctions is unknown. In some cases, the immune system attacks the thyroid, damaging and occasionally destroying it. Benign or malignant tumors can also form on the gland and render it useless. Infections can be a temporary interference to thyroid production.

Grave's Disease

Q: My daughter has Grave's disease. She's 20, was diagnosed two years ago. She's receiving medications, of course, but can she use any alternative medicines?

A: Grave's disease refers to an overactive thyroid, but the cause is unknown. It may be an autoimmune phenomenon, meaning the body starts to attack itself, producing antibodies that specifically affect the thyroid gland.

I would suggest that your daughter try to build up her immune system with astragalus. Unlike goldenseal and echinacea, astragalus can be taken for a period of time without becoming ineffective. I would also suggest that she take a good antioxidant to slow down her metabolism and lots of clean water. Chlorine mimics the sex hormone estrogen, so she should filter all her water before showering or using it for cooking.

> *To build up the immune system, try astragalus root.*

Your daughter could also benefit from eating the cruciferous vegetables such as broccoli and brussels sprouts as well as peaches, pears, soybeans, and spinach. She should not have stimulants containing caffeine, nor should she have alcohol or nicotine in any form.

Q: What is an antioxidant? I've never understood that.
A: Free radicals are produced in the metabolic process of oxidation. Free radicals don't have enough electrons attached to their oxygen molecules, so the oxygen molecules become very active and can do a lot of damage to your system.

Q: Isn't oxidation a basic process of metabolism?
A: Yes, it's a basic life process. You need the oxidative process to carry on life. But that oxidative process also produces toxins. So you don't want to stop oxidation, you want to stop the damage from the toxins it produces. Think of an iron pipe that's left outside. It rusts—it oxidizes. On its surface, iron molecules combine with oxygen molecules, and it becomes reddish brown. If you want to protect the pipe from rusting, you perhaps paint the surface so the damage can't occur.

In our bodies, we want to protect our systems from being damaged, too. Instead of painting, we keep oxygen molecules from damaging our system. Your daughter will benefit from these because her metabolism is speeding along at a high rate, and she's producing more free radicals than the average person. Counteract these with supplements such as coenzyme Q10, vitamin A, vitamin E, beta carotene, and vitamin C. All are excellent antioxidants. Follow the directions on all vitamins and supplements, especially the fat-soluble ones.

Q: What about grape-seed extract and pycnogenol? They're antioxidants, too.
A: Pycnogenol is actually a trade name for a particular brand of pinebark extract. Grape-seed extract is usually less expensive because grape seeds are more plentiful than pinebark. The active ingredients of both extracts are groups of flavonoids known as proanthocyanidolic oligomers or PCO. Grape-seed extracts have eighty-five to ninety-five percent PCO and pinebark extracts have eighty to eight-five percent. They are both excellent antioxidants. Does your daughter exercise?

Q: Yes, all the time.
A: Good. The only caution I would make is that she should work closely with her doctor to resolve her thyroid problem. If she marries and becomes pregnant, she again should be followed very closely by an endocrinologist.

The physical and hormonal changes that occur during pregnancy can require special monitoring.

Hypothyroidism

Q: Can hypothyroidism be helped with herbs? Before it was diagnosed, I was tired all the time and didn't want to eat, but I still gained a whole lot of weight. I had muscle cramps, too, and constipation. I thought I was losing my mind because I couldn't remember anything from one day to another. When I finally went to the doctor, he took some tests and found that my thyroid isn't working very well.

A: When you have a set of symptoms like that, you shouldn't delay going to the doctor. If your problems turn out to be minor, both you and your physician will be relieved. If your problem is more serious, you can begin prompt treatment. In the future, don't put off seeing your physician when things aren't right with you physically.

You can stimulate your thyroid gland with herbs. Iodine also protects the thyroid gland from radiation damage. Kelp contains iodine, so it's a useful dietary supplement for your condition, but kelp should not be used by anyone with a blood-pressure problem. You may also boost your immune system with goldenseal, taken only for seven days; black cohosh may also be useful.

As to your diet, drink only distilled water in order to avoid both the chlorine and fluoride that is usually added to the public water supply. Your diet should include parsley, apricots, and fish or chicken; avoid red meats, refined flour, sugar, and any kind of stimulant.

> *With a positive approach and persistence, you can lose weight.*

Thyroid and Weight Loss

Q: I'm concerned about my thyroid. My doctor says my thyroid tests show that it's normal, but I'm not sure. I'm 100 pounds overweight, and I feel like my thyroid must have something to do with it. I'm trying to lose weight and exercise, but it's awfully hard and time-consuming. I'm eating only 20 fat grams and 1,000 calories per day, and I'm miserable.

A: What kind of exercise are you doing?

Q: I try to swim a little once a week.

A: Swimming a little once a week with a diet of 1,000 calories per day is a great idea, but to lose weight and keep it off, you must build a habit of eating and exercising that you can sustain. Start slow—for the first week or two—then build your exercise to four days a week, then five days, then six. Over time you will come to enjoy it, and you will build a sustainable rate of weight loss that will become fairly consistent.

Your weight-loss goal ought not exceed two pounds per week. Losing a lot of weight fast, through frantic exercise and a very strict diet, usually leads to putting it back on. Building good eating and exercise habits, and sustaining them, leads to long-term, healthy weight loss.

There are a number of very successful weight-management programs sponsored by nonprofit organizations such as the American Heart Association. Your hospital may offer one, too. Commercial weight-loss programs, on the other hand, have a very low success rate, and they're very expensive.

Don't go for diet gimmicks such as breakfast shakes or diet pills. They just don't work over the long haul. The diet pills typically contain ephedra, which works as a stimulant, antihistamine, and bronchodilator. Ephedra wakes you up and relieves nasal and bronchial congestion, but unfortunately it also narrows the blood vessels and increases blood pressure. Men with prostate problems and anyone with high blood pressure should avoid these products. I advise my patients not to use any commercial preparation for weight loss, and if they feel they must, to be very cautious and never exceed the recommended dosage.

Don't overlook psychological and nutritional counseling. I've seen many people benefit from these approaches while they are struggling to lose weight. Weight loss is a difficult task, and I encourage my patients to find the support—all the *effective* support—that will help them succeed.

When my patients get discouraged about trying to lose weight, I remind them that every single person hospitalized for morbid obesity is given only a very limited number of calories in a balanced diet. These people succeed in losing weight. Anyone can do it, although it's difficult.

Hashimoto's Disease

Q: I've been diagnosed with Hashimoto's disease. I went to the doctor because I felt cold all the time and I gained a lot of weight, and it seemed like I just had no energy. What is this disease, anyway?

A: Hashimoto's disease is a disorder of the thyroid. We believe that the immune system attacks and damages the thyroid, making it ineffective and reducing or eliminating thyroid hormones available to maintain normal body functions. Because the thyroid regulates body temperature and energy output, it becomes impossible for you to stay warm when your surroundings are cold or even cool. You gain weight and feel lethargic because your body is not burning the calories for energy that it usually does. Typically, your thyroid gland is somewhat swollen, too.

This disorder usually develops over a long period of time. Because its symptoms can be related to a number of different disorders, it is best diagnosed by blood tests.

Q: Yes, my doctor said it's swollen. He didn't talk about surgery, but will I have to have that eventually?

A: Most cases of Hashimoto's disease respond quite well to treatment with various thyroid hormones, and surgery is unnecessary. With appropriate thyroid medication, you should feel better in two or three weeks, although you may need to continue the medication for a long time.

Diminished thyroid function can be very troublesome when it affects newborns. These children are at risk of dwarfism and mental retardation. Fortunately, newborns in most areas are routinely tested for this problem, and, with early diagnosis and treatment, the chances of the baby's having a normal life are very high. The problem can also become severe when it goes undiagnosed for a long period of time; the elderly are most frequently seen with severe undiagnosed thyroid dysfunction. Aggravating factors include sedatives, illness, exposure to cold, and traumas such as accident, injury, or surgery. At its most extreme, the dysfunction can cause confusion and life-threatening coma requiring emergency treatment. So it's a good thing that you went to the doctor when you did, thus avoiding possibility of severe problems.

Q: Are there any natural remedies to this disease?

A: You really need the medication that your physician prescribed for you. In addition, you can alter your diet by being sure that you purchase iodized salt for cooking and the table; iodine is the primary element that is missing from your system. Also add to your diet fish and chicken, molasses, and the stone fruits such as apricots and plums, fresh or dried. Exercise stimulates your thyroid function and is essential to regaining normal function. It will help you lose the extra weight, too.

Avoid the broccoli family of vegetables such as cabbage and brussels sprouts; also avoid spinach and peanuts in any form. Also, eliminate chlorine from your diet and your bath by filtering all the tap water that you use. Chlorine mimics some hormones, and you don't need that. Also, don't take antihistamines or antibiotics without your doctor's advice. Increase your intake of vitamin B complex vitamin B_{12}; you may also benefit from adding brewers yeast to your diet.

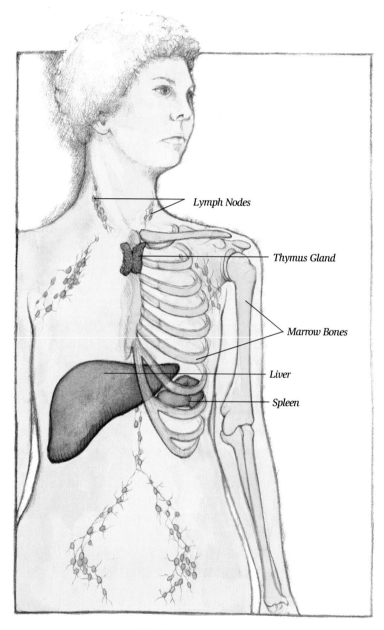

Lymph Nodes

Thymus Gland

Marrow Bones

Liver

Spleen

The Immune System

THE IMMUNE SYSTEM

*Preserving health is the normal function of the immune
system, but sometimes it goes awry.*

The immune system develops the idea of "self" for the body and
eliminates from the body all "nonself" elements such as microbes,
cancer cells, and toxins from the body. The immune system includes
the lymphatic system, the thymus gland, the spleen, the liver, white blood
cells, and special blood components. Each attacks different "nonself"
material. The liver, for instance, produces most of the lymphatic fluid in
the body. It also contains Kupffer cells that filter bacteria, candida, and
toxins from the gastrointestinal tract. No immune-system function is
effective alone; all act in concert to protect the body.

When the immune system is suppressed or damaged, illness and
disease easily develop. Worldwide, the most common cause of immune
suppression is malnutrition; infection inevitably follows starvation. An
ineffective immune system may be hereditary or result from exposure to
radiation, steroids, immunosuppressive drugs, or chemotherapy. Numerous
chronic illnesses such as leukemia, diabetes, and sickle-cell disease
suppress the immune system.

Confusion or dysfunction within the immune system may also cause
certain disorders. Researchers suspect that systemic lupus erythmatosus,
rheumatoid arthritis, and some cases of diabetes and infertility are related
to immune-system problems. In these cases, the immune system apparently fails to recognize essential components of the body as "self" and
attacks them, causing a deficiency. For instance, the pancreas's output of

insulin may be wrongly recognized as a foreign substance and destroyed; diabetes then occurs. Because the study of the immune system is relatively new, knowledge about it is developing rapidly, and many questions such as these have not been fully explored.

The function of immunity does not rest solely on the immune system. The skin protects against the entry of pathogens into the body and removes waste by perspiring. The digestive tract removes waste and excretes numerous pathogens. The respiratory tract and lungs are also essential in removing troublesome micro-organisms by capturing them in the mucous membranes and sweeping them, by means of the cilia cells, into the digestive tract, where they are destroyed. Only about ten percent of the microorganisms that enter the body actually reach the immune system.

With that fact in mind, overall health is a clear priority. When the skin, the digestive tract, and the respiratory tract perform well, the immune system usually is not overly stressed. If these support systems falter or decline, however, the immune system must carry a far greater load. The likelihood of it becoming overwhelmed, increases.

Stress, lack of refreshing sleep, and poor nutrition also work against the immune system. The high levels of catelochamines and adrenaline released when we feel stressed are intended only for short-term use in fight-or-flight situations. Unfortunately, most of us experience sustained levels of high stress, and excessive hormone secretions interfere with the immune system.

When stress is combined with disturbed sleep, as is common, the body cannot efficiently repair itself physically or mentally. Thus the individual faces a new day less able than before to deal effectively with more difficulties and stress. The immune system becomes more vulnerable.

Immune suppression resulting from poor nutrition is not only a third-world problem. Nearly two-thirds of our elderly are deficient in one or more nutritional elements, and many others have imbalanced diets. Without good nutrition, the immune system functions poorly.

FREQUENT INFECTIONS

Q: I seem to catch every cold and flu bug that goes around. Do you think

I should take some herbs for my immune system? What would help?
A: Several herbs are quite effective in counteracting these kinds of infection. The best known and most available immune-system stimulants are echinacea and goldenseal. Each can be taken as a tea, a tincture, or a powder.

Echinacea combats viruses by stimulating the white blood cells. It also interferes with the ability of viruses to reproduce and prevents them from attaching to the body's tissues. I tell my patients to take echinacea for one week only when they feel like they are coming down with something, and then to wait a week. If they still don't feel quite well, they should take echinacea for one more week. Echinacea taken continuously loses its effectiveness. And anyone who is allergic to echinacea's cousin ragweed should use the herb with caution.

Goldenseal is another herb that helps the immune system. It attacks microbes directly, and it also stimulates blood circulation to the spleen and activates the blood components that destroy bacteria and other dangerous invaders. Like echinacea, it should be taken for only a week at a time, and used cautiously by those allergic to sunflowers.

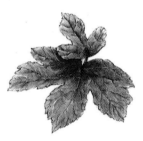

Several other herbs are effective in improving immunity. Astragalus can be used regularly; it stimulates the immune system's microbe-fighting cells and protects the adrenal glands. Astragalus is particularly aggressive against tumor cells, but should not be taken when fever is present. Licorice treats the respiratory tract and prevents viral infection; it also acts as an antibiotic. If you have high blood

goldenseal

pressure, make sure that your licorice is the deglycerrhizinated type, or DGL.

When you start to feel like you're getting sick, these herbs may prevent an illness or shorten its duration. Used carefully, they are very effective. You should visit your doctor promptly, however, when you have fever that is more than 101 degrees Fahrenheit or when your fever is accompanied by abdominal pain or a stiff neck. These symptoms can signal serious illness.

CHRONIC FATIGUE SYNDROME

Q: Can herbs help chronic fatigue syndrome?

A: It is estimated that half a million people in the United States suffer from chronic fatigue syndrome. In 1988, the National Center for Disease Control established clear criteria to define the illness, but medical records since the 1860s have described the syndrome under many different names. To be diagnosed with CFS, the patient must have each of the following symptoms:

1. A new onset of fatigue reducing activity by fifty percent or more and lasting for at least six months.
2. Exclusion of other illnesses that can cause fatigue.

The patient must also report at least four of the following symptoms:

    a. Neurological or psychological difficulties such as forgetfulness, confusion, impaired concentration, irritability, or depression.

    b. Recurring sore throat

    c. Painful lymph nodes

    d. Muscle pain and/or weakness

    e. Pain in multiple joints

    f. Recurrent new headaches

    g. Disturbed sleep

    h. Post-exertion malaise

Finally, tests must exclude the possibility of hepatitis, diabetes, cancer, liver disease, depression, and other ailments that have symptoms similar to chronic fatigue syndrome. Less than five percent of people who claim persistent fatigue fit the criteria, so "chronic fatigue" sometimes becomes a catch-all term for feeling tired.

Some people complain that the testing for other ailments is useless, but I disagree. If I were to presume that a patient has chronic fatigue syndrome and prescribe for it without being sure, the patient would not improve. If, in fact, the symptoms are caused by a malfunctioning thyroid, then astragalus, echinacea, and vitamins won't help. It's important to rule out other disorders in the process of diagnosing chronic fatigue syndrome.

When the diagnosis of chronic fatigue is firm, vitamins A, E, and C can be used as antioxidants and energy boosters. Ginkgo biloba increases mental alertness by stimulating circulation to the brain. If infection threatens, use goldenseal or echinacea. It's good to carefully monitor the blood pressure, too, as some who suffer from CFS have low blood pressure and can benefit from treatment for it.

Add acidophilus to a diet that includes plenty of fiber, clean, filtered water, and fresh vegetables. Many CFS patients have overgrowths of candida and improve when this is brought under control, so removing refined flour and all forms of sugar from the diet can be very useful. Adequate sleep is essential, too.

Q: My mother-in-law was diagnosed with Epstein-Barr virus (EBV) some time ago. Isn't that the same as chronic fatigue syndrome?
A: Epstein-Barr virus, a member of the herpes group, may be related to CFS but we don't understand the connection. Like other herpes types, EBV can hide itself in the body after the initial infection and remain inactive for long periods. But a number of other infectious organisms are also suspected as agents of CFS.

We do know that sixty percent of people with EBV also have yeast problems. Acidophilus, then, is very important in their treatment.

Q: Somebody told me recently that if you have chronic fatigue syndrome, you get better after some six or eight years.
A: I've heard that, too, but I don't know that it is true. It may be that as people with CFS are carefully examined over a long period of time—and this hasn't been done before—we will find that there is a time when this illness resolves. Perhaps it has a life cycle of its own. But we must wait for the results of research to know for sure.

Chronic Fatigue and Infection
Q: My cousin has chronic fatigue syndrome. Last summer she had a severe stomach infection, and afterwards she was diagnosed as having chronic fatigue syndrome. Do you think there's a relationship between the two?
A: I can't really say for sure without knowing more about the stomach infection. If she has chronic fatigue syndrome, however, she may well have an overgrowth of candida in her system. I tell my patients with chronic fatigue syndrome to take the sugar and refined flour out of their diet and start taking acidophilus. Many find that the fatigue begins to

disappear soon after they make this change.

Q: So for someone who has fibromyalgia, could reading The Yeast Connection *and following that diet be good?*
A: It would be excellent! While fibromyalgia and chronic fatigue syndrome are entirely different illnesses, I've had patients with each that have responded positively to controlling candida with acidophilus.

In my own practice, I often find a white coating on a patient's tongue, usually so thick that I can't see the papillae. Of course these patients report that their food tastes different, and they have problems with bad breath. That coating is typically candida, and if it has reached the tongue, it's all the way through the digestive tract. I prescribe a few days' worth of antifungal medication to accompany a diet that emphasizes raw foods and fresh juices along with whole grains, nuts and seeds, plus a little turkey and fish. Using acidophilus is also important. It takes at least six weeks for the acidophilus to work, and then we begin to see healing.

LUPUS

Q: Several of my acquaintances have recently been diagnosed with lupus. It seems to affect each of them quite differently.
A: Lupus is an inflammation of the connective tissue, which is found throughout the body. That's why individuals can demonstrate so many different symptoms. There are two basic types of lupus. Discoid lupus erythematosus (DLE) is chronic and confined to the skin. Although this lupus is disfiguring and painful, it generally is not life-threatening. The second type, systemic lupus erythematosus (SLE), can range from mild to severe and involve numerous organs. Women suffer ninety percent of the lupus cases, and those of Asian heritage are more likely than others to get it. The cause of lupus is unknown, but many strongly suspect an immune-system dysfunction in which the system attacks the body's connective tissues. Viral or environmental triggers may also play a role.

Lupus may begin with vague aches and pains that resemble those of arthritis, or it can strike suddenly with a high fever. Patients with both types can develop a persistent, symmetrical butterfly-shaped rash on the cheeks. This and other lupus symptoms may come and go, sometimes staying in remission for years, at other times persisting for long periods. The course of the disease is completely unpredictable. It is typically treated symptomatically; severe cases are treated with prednisone.

Q: Does lupus have complications?
A: The different ways that lupus affects people make it seem like it has complications. People with lupus often come to the doctor thinking that they have arthritis because their joints are swollen, red, and inflamed, and they are surprised to find that they have lupus. Inflammation of the kidney is another common symptom that can become quite serious if not treated conscientiously. The lungs are also frequently attacked by lupus. The central nervous system, including the brain, may become involved in severe cases, leading to seizures, deep depression, and psychosis.

Fortunately, the pattern of lupus is one of flare-up and remission. Many who suffer from the disorder may find that by avoiding bright sunlight, fatigue, and stress, they find relief from symptoms. Other factors that may contribute to increased symptoms of lupus are pregnancy and childbirth, viral or bacterial infection, medications, and exposure to chemicals. These symptoms are highly individual, however.

Q: Are there any natural medicines that help people with lupus?
A: Herbs can help support the body and heal it during lupus flare-ups. Because the skin is so often involved, a clean intestine and excellent digestion are important, so lots of fiber, fruit and vegetables, plus supplements of acidophilus may be helpful. Also eliminate red meat, dairy products, refined flour products, and citrus fruits. Antioxidants such as grape-seed extract, vitamin A, and vitamin E help protect the body from damage. Milk thistle protects the liver, which is often attacked by lupus. Determining which herbs and supplements will be helpful depends on the individual's symptoms.

Avoid herbs that strengthen the immune system if you have lupus.

Take care to avoid echinacea, goldenseal, and astragalus if you have lupus or another illness that is caused by an overactive or misdirected immune system. Strengthening the immune system with these herbs may encourage the immune system to damage the body to a greater degree.

ANTIBIOTICS AND IMMUNITY

Q: Is it true that antibiotics undermine the immune system and predispose us to infections?
A: We target certain infectious bacteria when selecting penicillin, tetracycline, or another antibiotic for a given problem. The antibiotic's action usually kills the target bacteria, but, unfortunately, it kills beneficial bacteria as well. The result is often the overgrowth of the yeast candida. That's why I recommend taking acidophilus—to replace the good bacteria destroyed by the antibiotic, and to prevent the growth of too much candida.

Q: But do antibiotics impair the immune system?
A: Just as you can be allergic to tomatoes, you can be allergic to tetracycline; any individual can develop an allergy to almost any substance. Certain people are allergic to antibiotics, most often to penicillin, but otherwise antibiotics don't depress, destroy, or otherwise damage the immune system. In fact, antibiotics are sometimes necessary to help the immune system overcome severe infections like staphylococcus.

Q: If I take antibiotics, am I more susceptible to disease?
A: If you are taking the right antibiotic for your condition, in the right amount, no. In fact, your health will be improved.

Broadly, however, doctors and patients alike must rethink how we prescribe and take antibiotics because new drug-resistant strains of serious disease have developed. Not so long ago, we believed that the new antibiotics were wonderful and would protect us eternally against illness, so they were prescribed often, whether the patient's condition warranted them or not. We were prescribing antibiotics when they were effective, but we were also prescribing them inappropriately to cure viral infections or to protect against possible infection. And, we thought, if one round of antibiotic didn't cure the problem, maybe two or three would.

Patients, for their part, were taking antibiotics only until they felt better, ignoring the fact that an incomplete course of the medication would not eliminate the infection. Some patients hoarded their drugs, saving some for later infections. When they did get sick again, they took another few antibiotics until the symptoms eased—that is, until the infection was knocked down, but not out.